EXCELLENCE IN TRAINING

A Race Walking Specific Training Log

Caitlin,
I am very impressed with the progress you have made so far but I am super excited about what the future results will be. Keep up the good work,
Tim Seaman

By Jeff Salvage

&

Tim Seaman

Caitlin,
You style is great. Keep up the good work & you'll be winning everything you enter.
Jeff Salvage

Caitlin,
You have so much talent! Keep working on your technique and keep training smart. You have the ability to be on a USA team. Dream big! Best of luck!
Rachel Seaman
Canadian Champion

79 North Lakeside Drive W

Medford, NJ 08055

This book is dedicated to two wonderful, contemporary contributors to the world of race walking. Without their unwavering support our sport would be significantly smaller and less accomplished:

Tom Eastler & A.C. Jaime

INTRODUCTION

We all know we should keep a training log. It allows you to keep track of your successes and perhaps more importantly, learn from your mistakes. Some of us scribble down our workouts in an inconsistent manner, while many of us do not get beyond the new season's resolution to keep better track of our workouts. Now with *Excellence in Training – A Race Walking Specific Training Log*, you have a simple template-based system to record all of the pertinent details of your training and hopefully be inspired along the way. Our template includes space for you to record your workouts for 52 weeks of the year as well as photographs of some of the best race walkers in the world achieving the speeds we aspire to.

Our training log is based on two-time Olympian Tim Seaman's personal training log. It's one that he perfected over a career that includes 38 US National titles. The log contains room for you to record workouts 7 days a week for 52 weeks of the year. There is space allowing you to record many specific aspects of your daily training as well as containing an area for more general notes each day. In addition, each week contains an area for any other notes that might not be captured within the template. At the end of the log, we include space for monthly totals, race results, and a personal records (PRs) progression. So take a step into a champion's shoes and start your progression to a more successful walking program by filling out your training log today.

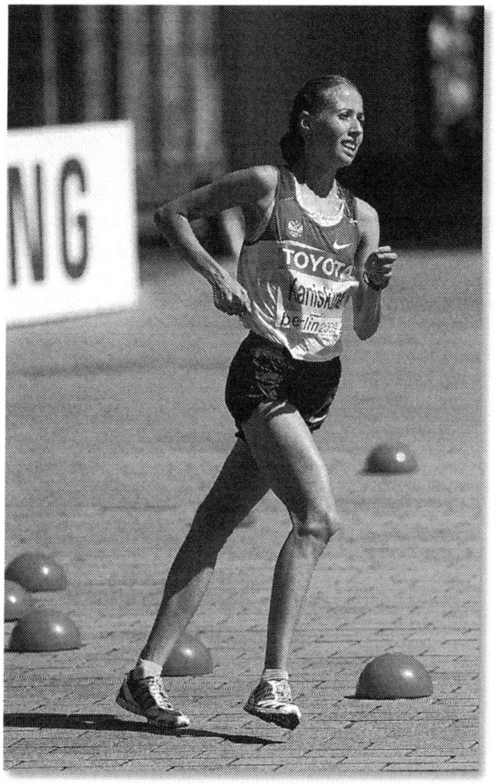

Olga Kaniskina - Russia
Olympic and two time World Champion
20km PR: 1:24:56

Weekly Notes

MONDAY

TUESDAY

WEDNESDAY

THURSDAY

FRIDAY

SATURDAY

SUNDAY

MONDAY	Date:	Location:	2nd workout:
W/U Distance :	W/U Time:		
Workout Type:			
C/D Distance:	C/D Time:	Total Daily Distance:	

TUESDAY	Date:	Location:	2nd workout:
W/U Distance :	W/U Time:		
Workout Type:			
C/D Distance:	C/D Time:	Total Daily Distance:	

WEDNESDAY	Date:	Location:	2nd workout:
W/U Distance :	W/U Time:		
Workout Type:			
C/D Distance:	C/D Time:	Total Daily Distance:	

THURSDAY	Date:	Location:	2nd workout:
W/U Distance :	W/U Time:		
Workout Type:			
C/D Distance:	C/D Time:	Total Daily Distance:	

FRIDAY	Date:	Location:	2nd workout:
W/U Distance :	W/U Time:		
Workout Type:			
C/D Distance:	C/D Time:	Total Daily Distance:	

SATURDAY	Date:	Location:	2nd workout:
W/U Distance :	W/U Time:		
Workout Type:			
C/D Distance:	C/D Time:	Total Daily Distance:	

SUNDAY	Date:	Location:	2nd workout:
W/U Distance :	W/U Time:		
Workout Type:			
C/D Distance:	C/D Time:	Total Daily Distance:	

Total Distance for the Week:	

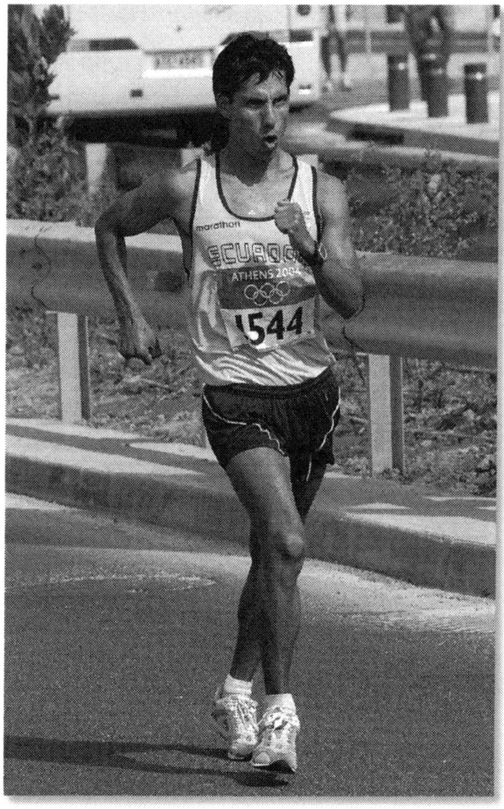

Jefferson Perez – Ecuador
20km PR: 1:17:21, 50km PR:3:53:04
Three Time World Champion
Olympic Gold and Silver Medalist
Former World Record Holder

Weekly Notes

MONDAY

TUESDAY

WEDNESDAY

THURSDAY

FRIDAY

SATURDAY

SUNDAY

MONDAY	Date:	Location:	2nd workout:
W/U Distance :	W/U Time:		
Workout Type:			Total Daily Distance:
C/D Distance:	C/D Time:		

TUESDAY	Date:	Location:	2nd workout:
W/U Distance :	W/U Time:		
Workout Type:			Total Daily Distance:
C/D Distance:	C/D Time:		

WEDNESDAY	Date:	Location:	2nd workout:
W/U Distance :	W/U Time:		
Workout Type:			Total Daily Distance:
C/D Distance:	C/D Time:		

THURSDAY	Date:	Location:	2nd workout:
W/U Distance :	W/U Time:		
Workout Type:			Total Daily Distance:
C/D Distance:	C/D Time:		

FRIDAY	Date:	Location:	2nd workout:
W/U Distance :	W/U Time:		
Workout Type:			Total Daily Distance:
C/D Distance:	C/D Time:		

SATURDAY	Date:	Location:	2nd workout:
W/U Distance :	W/U Time:		
Workout Type:			Total Daily Distance:
C/D Distance:	C/D Time:		

SUNDAY	Date:	Location:	2nd workout:
W/U Distance :	W/U Time:		
Workout Type:			Total Daily Distance:
C/D Distance:	C/D Time:		

Total Distance for the Week:	

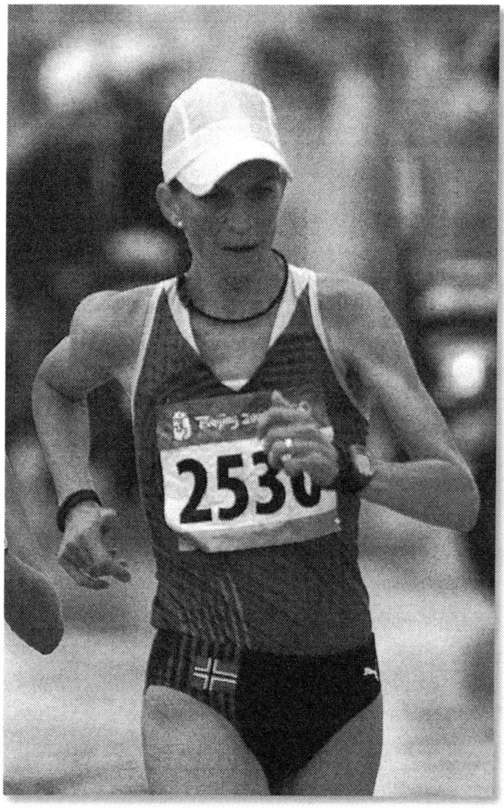

Kjersti Plätzer – Norway
20km PR: 1:27:07
Two time silver medalist – Olympic Games

Weekly Notes

MONDAY

TUESDAY

WEDNESDAY

THURSDAY

FRIDAY

SATURDAY

SUNDAY

MONDAY	Date:	Location:	2nd workout:
W/U Distance :		W/U Time:	
Workout Type:			Total Daily Distance:
C/D Distance:		C/D Time:	

TUESDAY	Date:	Location:	2nd workout:
W/U Distance :		W/U Time:	
Workout Type:			Total Daily Distance:
C/D Distance:		C/D Time:	

WEDNESDAY	Date:	Location:	2nd workout:
W/U Distance :		W/U Time:	
Workout Type:			Total Daily Distance:
C/D Distance:		C/D Time:	

THURSDAY	Date:	Location:	2nd workout:
W/U Distance :		W/U Time:	
Workout Type:			Total Daily Distance:
C/D Distance:		C/D Time:	

FRIDAY	Date:	Location:	2nd workout:
W/U Distance :		W/U Time:	
Workout Type:			Total Daily Distance:
C/D Distance:		C/D Time:	

SATURDAY	Date:	Location:	2nd workout:
W/U Distance :		W/U Time:	
Workout Type:			Total Daily Distance:
C/D Distance:		C/D Time:	

SUNDAY	Date:	Location:	2nd workout:
W/U Distance :		W/U Time:	
Workout Type:			Total Daily Distance:
C/D Distance:		C/D Time:	

	Total Distance for the Week:	

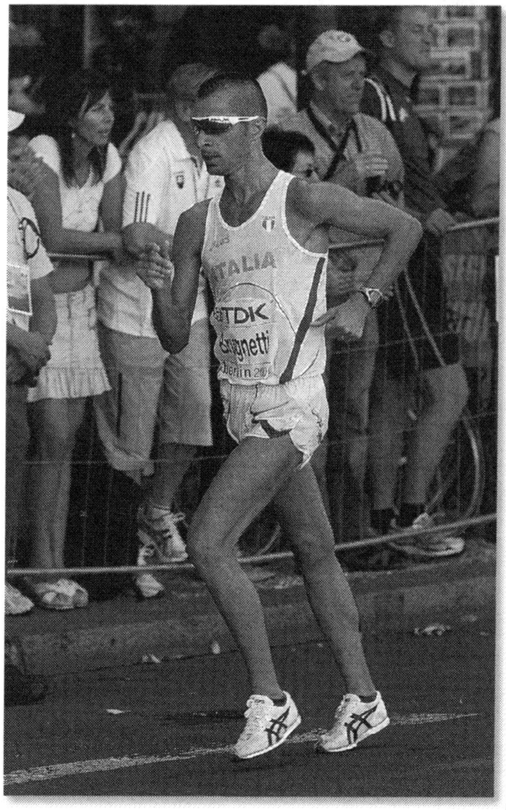

Ivano Brugnetti – Italy
20km PR: 1:19:36, 50km PR: 3:47:54
World and Olympic Champion

<u>Weekly Notes</u>

MONDAY
TUESDAY
WEDNESDAY
THURSDAY
FRIDAY
SATURDAY
SUNDAY

MONDAY	Date:	Location:	2nd workout:
W/U Distance :	W/U Time:		
Workout Type:			Total Daily Distance:
C/D Distance:	C/D Time:		

TUESDAY	Date:	Location:	2nd workout:
W/U Distance :	W/U Time:		
Workout Type:			Total Daily Distance:
C/D Distance:	C/D Time:		

WEDNESDAY	Date:	Location:	2nd workout:
W/U Distance :	W/U Time:		
Workout Type:			Total Daily Distance:
C/D Distance:	C/D Time:		

THURSDAY	Date:	Location:	2nd workout:
W/U Distance :	W/U Time:		
Workout Type:			Total Daily Distance:
C/D Distance:	C/D Time:		

FRIDAY	Date:	Location:	2nd workout:
W/U Distance :	W/U Time:		
Workout Type:			Total Daily Distance:
C/D Distance:	C/D Time:		

SATURDAY	Date:	Location:	2nd workout:
W/U Distance :	W/U Time:		
Workout Type:			Total Daily Distance:
C/D Distance:	C/D Time:		

SUNDAY	Date:	Location:	2nd workout:
W/U Distance :	W/U Time:		
Workout Type:			Total Daily Distance:
C/D Distance:	C/D Time:		

Total Distance for the Week:	

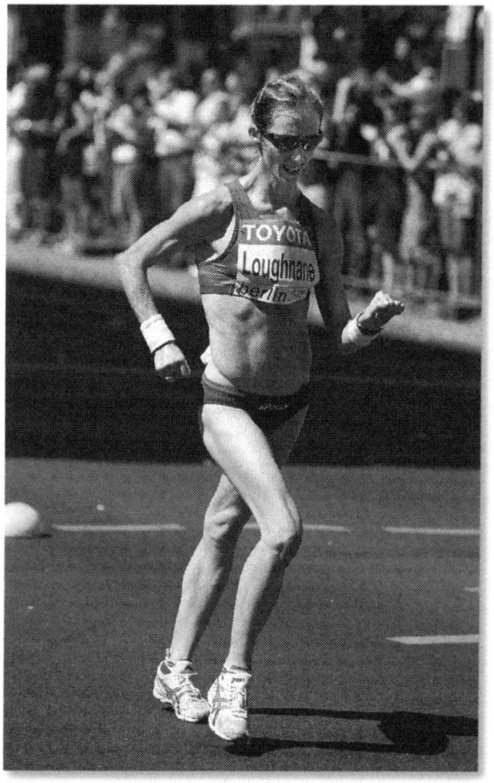

Olive Loughnane – Ireland
20km PR: 1:27:45
World Championships Silver Medalist

Weekly Notes

MONDAY

TUESDAY

WEDNESDAY

THURSDAY

FRIDAY

SATURDAY

SUNDAY

MONDAY	Date:	Location:	2nd workout:
W/U Distance :	W/U Time:		
Workout Type:			Total Daily Distance:
C/D Distance:	C/D Time:		

TUESDAY	Date:	Location:	2nd workout:
W/U Distance :	W/U Time:		
Workout Type:			Total Daily Distance:
C/D Distance:	C/D Time:		

WEDNESDAY	Date:	Location:	2nd workout:
W/U Distance :	W/U Time:		
Workout Type:			Total Daily Distance:
C/D Distance:	C/D Time:		

THURSDAY	Date:	Location:	2nd workout:
W/U Distance :	W/U Time:		
Workout Type:			Total Daily Distance:
C/D Distance:	C/D Time:		

FRIDAY	Date:	Location:	2nd workout:
W/U Distance :	W/U Time:		
Workout Type:			Total Daily Distance:
C/D Distance:	C/D Time:		

SATURDAY	Date:	Location:	2nd workout:
W/U Distance :	W/U Time:		
Workout Type:			Total Daily Distance:
C/D Distance:	C/D Time:		

SUNDAY	Date:	Location:	2nd workout:
W/U Distance :	W/U Time:		
Workout Type:			Total Daily Distance:
C/D Distance:	C/D Time:		

Total Distance for the Week:	

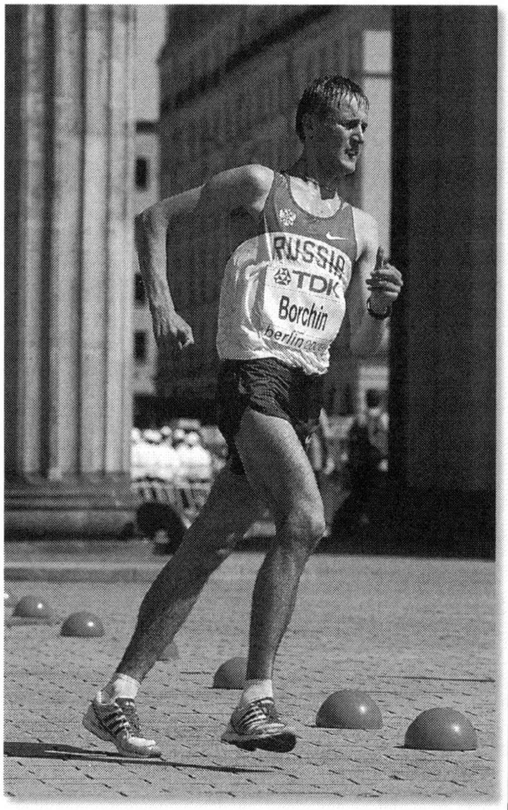

Valeriy Borchin – Russia
20km PR: 1:17:38
World and Olympic Champion

MONDAY

TUESDAY

WEDNESDAY

THURSDAY

FRIDAY

SATURDAY

SUNDAY

Weekly Notes

MONDAY	Date:	Location:	2nd workout:
W/U Distance :	W/U Time:		
Workout Type:			Total Daily Distance:
C/D Distance:	C/D Time:		

TUESDAY	Date:	Location:	2nd workout:
W/U Distance :	W/U Time:		
Workout Type:			Total Daily Distance:
C/D Distance:	C/D Time:		

WEDNESDAY	Date:	Location:	2nd workout:
W/U Distance :	W/U Time:		
Workout Type:			Total Daily Distance:
C/D Distance:	C/D Time:		

THURSDAY	Date:	Location:	2nd workout:
W/U Distance :	W/U Time:		
Workout Type:			Total Daily Distance:
C/D Distance:	C/D Time:		

FRIDAY	Date:	Location:	2nd workout:
W/U Distance :	W/U Time:		
Workout Type:			Total Daily Distance:
C/D Distance:	C/D Time:		

SATURDAY	Date:	Location:	2nd workout:
W/U Distance :	W/U Time:		
Workout Type:			Total Daily Distance:
C/D Distance:	C/D Time:		

SUNDAY	Date:	Location:	2nd workout:
W/U Distance :	W/U Time:		
Workout Type:			Total Daily Distance:
C/D Distance:	C/D Time:		

Total Distance for the Week:	

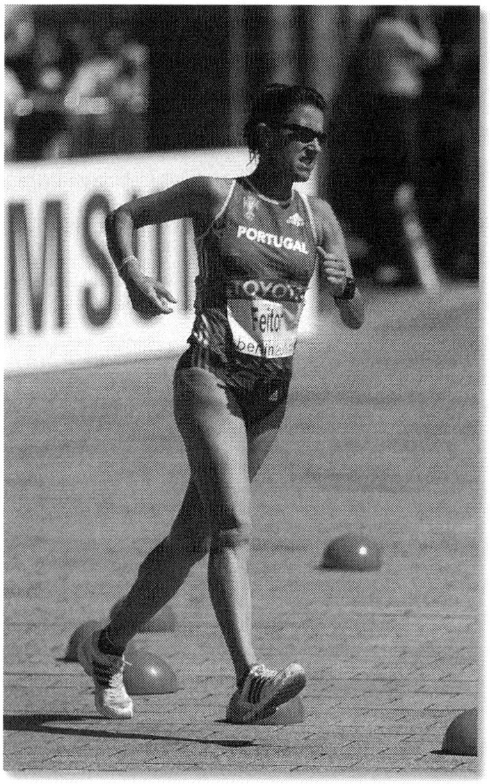

Susana Feitor – Portugal
20km PR: 1:27:55
World Championships Bronze Medalist
Five time Olympian

Weekly Notes

MONDAY

TUESDAY

WEDNESDAY

THURSDAY

FRIDAY

SATURDAY

SUNDAY

MONDAY	Date:	Location:	2nd workout:
W/U Distance :	W/U Time:		
Workout Type:			Total Daily Distance:
C/D Distance:	C/D Time:		

TUESDAY	Date:	Location:	2nd workout:
W/U Distance :	W/U Time:		
Workout Type:			Total Daily Distance:
C/D Distance:	C/D Time:		

WEDNESDAY	Date:	Location:	2nd workout:
W/U Distance :	W/U Time:		
Workout Type:			Total Daily Distance:
C/D Distance:	C/D Time:		

THURSDAY	Date:	Location:	2nd workout:
W/U Distance :	W/U Time:		
Workout Type:			Total Daily Distance:
C/D Distance:	C/D Time:		

FRIDAY	Date:	Location:	2nd workout:
W/U Distance :	W/U Time:		
Workout Type:			Total Daily Distance:
C/D Distance:	C/D Time:		

SATURDAY	Date:	Location:	2nd workout:
W/U Distance :	W/U Time:		
Workout Type:			Total Daily Distance:
C/D Distance:	C/D Time:		

SUNDAY	Date:	Location:	2nd workout:
W/U Distance :	W/U Time:		
Workout Type:			Total Daily Distance:
C/D Distance:	C/D Time:		

Total Distance for the Week:	

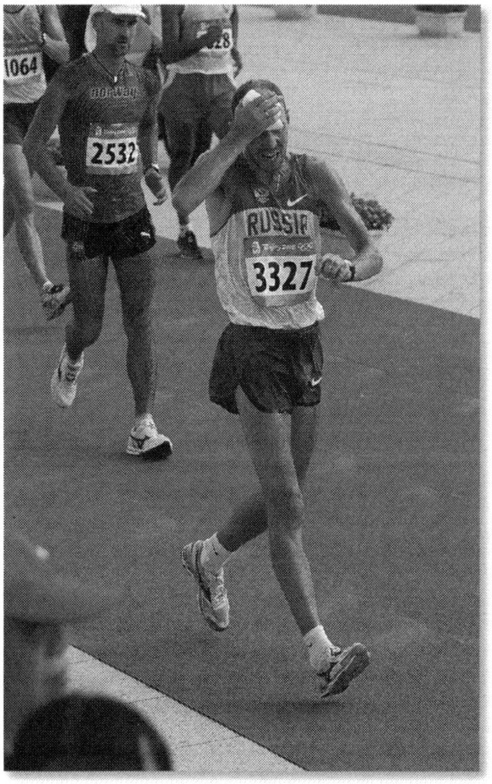

Sergey Kirdyapkin – Russia
20km PR: 1:23:24, 50km PR: 3:38:08
Two Time World Champion

Weekly Notes

MONDAY
TUESDAY
WEDNESDAY
THURSDAY
FRIDAY
SATURDAY
SUNDAY

MONDAY	Date:	Location:	2nd workout:	
W/U Distance :		W/U Time:		
Workout Type:				
C/D Distance:		C/D Time:	Total Daily Distance:	

TUESDAY	Date:	Location:	2nd workout:	
W/U Distance :		W/U Time:		
Workout Type:				
C/D Distance:		C/D Time:	Total Daily Distance:	

WEDNESDAY	Date:	Location:	2nd workout:	
W/U Distance :		W/U Time:		
Workout Type:				
C/D Distance:		C/D Time:	Total Daily Distance:	

THURSDAY	Date:	Location:	2nd workout:	
W/U Distance :		W/U Time:		
Workout Type:				
C/D Distance:		C/D Time:	Total Daily Distance:	

FRIDAY	Date:	Location:	2nd workout:	
W/U Distance :		W/U Time:		
Workout Type:				
C/D Distance:		C/D Time:	Total Daily Distance:	

SATURDAY	Date:	Location:	2nd workout:	
W/U Distance :		W/U Time:		
Workout Type:				
C/D Distance:		C/D Time:	Total Daily Distance:	

SUNDAY	Date:	Location:	2nd workout:	
W/U Distance :		W/U Time:		
Workout Type:				
C/D Distance:		C/D Time:	Total Daily Distance:	

Total Distance for the Week:	

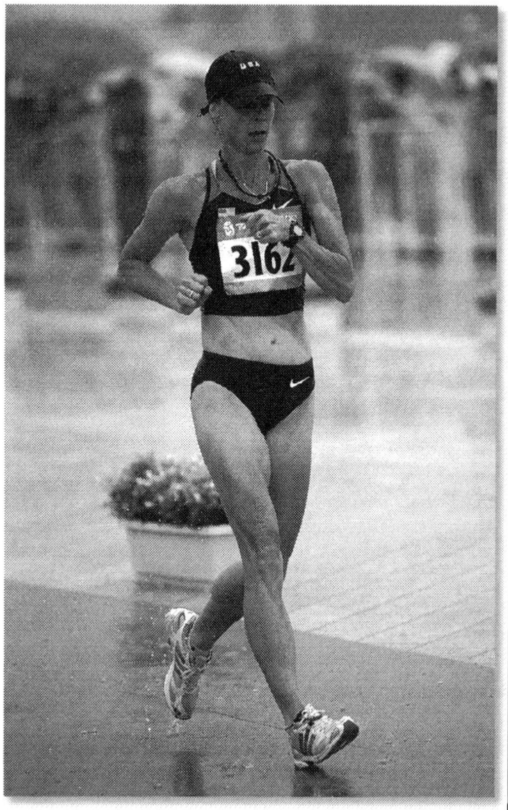

Joanne Dow – USA
20km PR: 1:32:54
Olympian

Weekly Notes

MONDAY

TUESDAY

WEDNESDAY

THURSDAY

FRIDAY

SATURDAY

SUNDAY

MONDAY	Date:	Location:	2nd workout:	
W/U Distance :	W/U Time:			
Workout Type:			Total Daily Distance:	
C/D Distance:	C/D Time:			
TUESDAY	Date:	Location:	2nd workout:	
W/U Distance :	W/U Time:			
Workout Type:			Total Daily Distance:	
C/D Distance:	C/D Time:			
WEDNESDAY	Date:	Location:	2nd workout:	
W/U Distance :	W/U Time:			
Workout Type:			Total Daily Distance:	
C/D Distance:	C/D Time:			
THURSDAY	Date:	Location:	2nd workout:	
W/U Distance :	W/U Time:			
Workout Type:			Total Daily Distance:	
C/D Distance:	C/D Time:			
FRIDAY	Date:	Location:	2nd workout:	
W/U Distance :	W/U Time:			
Workout Type:			Total Daily Distance:	
C/D Distance:	C/D Time:			
SATURDAY	Date:	Location:	2nd workout:	
W/U Distance :	W/U Time:			
Workout Type:			Total Daily Distance:	
C/D Distance:	C/D Time:			
SUNDAY	Date:	Location:	2nd workout:	
W/U Distance :	W/U Time:			
Workout Type:			Total Daily Distance:	
C/D Distance:	C/D Time:			
		Total Distance for the Week:		

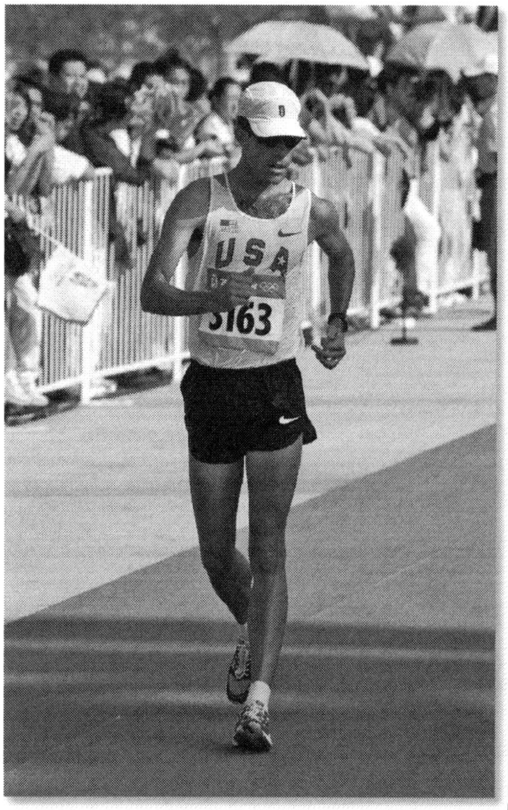

Philip Dunn – USA
20km PR: 1:26:36, 50km PR:3:56:13
Three Time Olympian

Weekly Notes

MONDAY

TUESDAY

WEDNESDAY

THURSDAY

FRIDAY

SATURDAY

SUNDAY

MONDAY	Date:	Location:	2nd workout:	
W/U Distance :		W/U Time:		
Workout Type:				
C/D Distance:		C/D Time:	Total Daily Distance:	

TUESDAY	Date:	Location:	2nd workout:	
W/U Distance :		W/U Time:		
Workout Type:				
C/D Distance:		C/D Time:	Total Daily Distance:	

WEDNESDAY	Date:	Location:	2nd workout:	
W/U Distance :		W/U Time:		
Workout Type:				
C/D Distance:		C/D Time:	Total Daily Distance:	

THURSDAY	Date:	Location:	2nd workout:	
W/U Distance :		W/U Time:		
Workout Type:				
C/D Distance:		C/D Time:	Total Daily Distance:	

FRIDAY	Date:	Location:	2nd workout:	
W/U Distance :		W/U Time:		
Workout Type:				
C/D Distance:		C/D Time:	Total Daily Distance:	

SATURDAY	Date:	Location:	2nd workout:	
W/U Distance :		W/U Time:		
Workout Type:				
C/D Distance:		C/D Time:	Total Daily Distance:	

SUNDAY	Date:	Location:	2nd workout:	
W/U Distance :		W/U Time:		
Workout Type:				
C/D Distance:		C/D Time:	Total Daily Distance:	

Total Distance for the Week:	

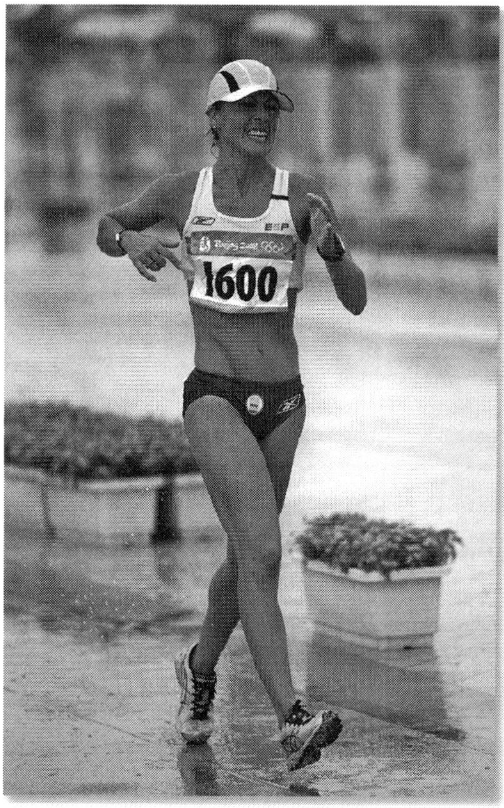

Maria Vasco – Spain
20km PR: 1:27:25
Bronze Medalist – Olympic Games, World Championships, & World Cup

Weekly Notes

MONDAY
TUESDAY
WEDNESDAY
THURSDAY
FRIDAY
SATURDAY
SUNDAY

MONDAY	**Date:**	**Location:**	**2nd workout:**
W/U Distance :	**W/U Time:**		
Workout Type:			**Total Daily Distance:**
C/D Distance:	**C/D Time:**		

TUESDAY	**Date:**	**Location:**	**2nd workout:**
W/U Distance :	**W/U Time:**		
Workout Type:			**Total Daily Distance:**
C/D Distance:	**C/D Time:**		

WEDNESDAY	**Date:**	**Location:**	**2nd workout:**
W/U Distance :	**W/U Time:**		
Workout Type:			**Total Daily Distance:**
C/D Distance:	**C/D Time:**		

THURSDAY	**Date:**	**Location:**	**2nd workout:**
W/U Distance :	**W/U Time:**		
Workout Type:			**Total Daily Distance:**
C/D Distance:	**C/D Time:**		

FRIDAY	**Date:**	**Location:**	**2nd workout:**
W/U Distance :	**W/U Time:**		
Workout Type:			**Total Daily Distance:**
C/D Distance:	**C/D Time:**		

SATURDAY	**Date:**	**Location:**	**2nd workout:**
W/U Distance :	**W/U Time:**		
Workout Type:			**Total Daily Distance:**
C/D Distance:	**C/D Time:**		

SUNDAY	**Date:**	**Location:**	**2nd workout:**
W/U Distance :	**W/U Time:**		
Workout Type:			**Total Daily Distance:**
C/D Distance:	**C/D Time:**		

Total Distance for the Week:	

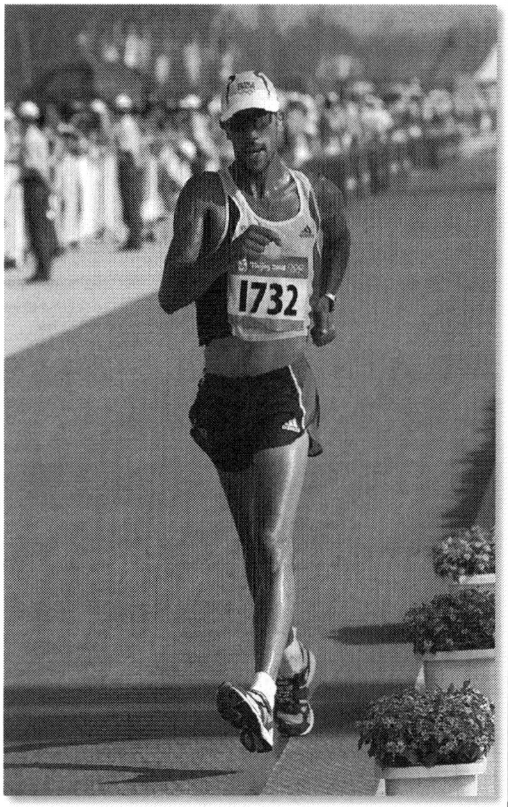

Yohan Diniz – France
20km PR: 1:18:58, 50km PR: 3:38:45
World Championships Silver Medalist

Weekly Notes

MONDAY

TUESDAY

WEDNESDAY

THURSDAY

FRIDAY

SATURDAY

SUNDAY

MONDAY	**Date:**	**Location:**	**2nd workout:**
W/U Distance :	**W/U Time:**		
Workout Type:			**Total Daily Distance:**
C/D Distance:	**C/D Time:**		
TUESDAY	**Date:**	**Location:**	**2nd workout:**
W/U Distance :	**W/U Time:**		
Workout Type:			**Total Daily Distance:**
C/D Distance:	**C/D Time:**		
WEDNESDAY	**Date:**	**Location:**	**2nd workout:**
W/U Distance :	**W/U Time:**		
Workout Type:			**Total Daily Distance:**
C/D Distance:	**C/D Time:**		
THURSDAY	**Date:**	**Location:**	**2nd workout:**
W/U Distance :	**W/U Time:**		
Workout Type:			**Total Daily Distance:**
C/D Distance:	**C/D Time:**		
FRIDAY	**Date:**	**Location:**	**2nd workout:**
W/U Distance :	**W/U Time:**		
Workout Type:			**Total Daily Distance:**
C/D Distance:	**C/D Time:**		
SATURDAY	**Date:**	**Location:**	**2nd workout:**
W/U Distance :	**W/U Time:**		
Workout Type:			**Total Daily Distance:**
C/D Distance:	**C/D Time:**		
SUNDAY	**Date:**	**Location:**	**2nd workout:**
W/U Distance :	**W/U Time:**		
Workout Type:			**Total Daily Distance:**
C/D Distance:	**C/D Time:**		
		Total Distance for the Week:	

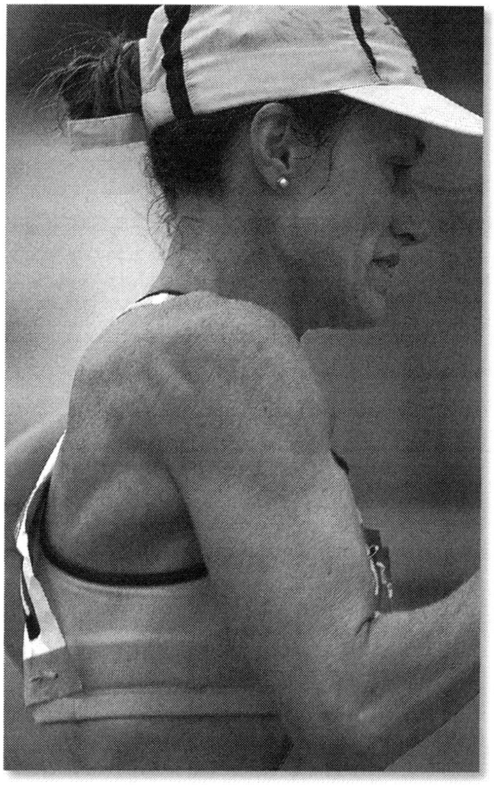

Jane Sayville – Australia
20km PR: 1:27:44
Olympic Bronze Medalist

Weekly Notes

MONDAY

TUESDAY

WEDNESDAY

THURSDAY

FRIDAY

SATURDAY

SUNDAY

MONDAY	Date:	Location:	2nd workout:
W/U Distance :		W/U Time:	
Workout Type:			Total Daily Distance:
C/D Distance:		C/D Time:	

TUESDAY	Date:	Location:	2nd workout:
W/U Distance :		W/U Time:	
Workout Type:			Total Daily Distance:
C/D Distance:		C/D Time:	

WEDNESDAY	Date:	Location:	2nd workout:
W/U Distance :		W/U Time:	
Workout Type:			Total Daily Distance:
C/D Distance:		C/D Time:	

THURSDAY	Date:	Location:	2nd workout:
W/U Distance :		W/U Time:	
Workout Type:			Total Daily Distance:
C/D Distance:		C/D Time:	

FRIDAY	Date:	Location:	2nd workout:
W/U Distance :		W/U Time:	
Workout Type:			Total Daily Distance:
C/D Distance:		C/D Time:	

SATURDAY	Date:	Location:	2nd workout:
W/U Distance :		W/U Time:	
Workout Type:			Total Daily Distance:
C/D Distance:		C/D Time:	

SUNDAY	Date:	Location:	2nd workout:
W/U Distance :		W/U Time:	
Workout Type:			Total Daily Distance:
C/D Distance:		C/D Time:	

Total Distance for the Week:	

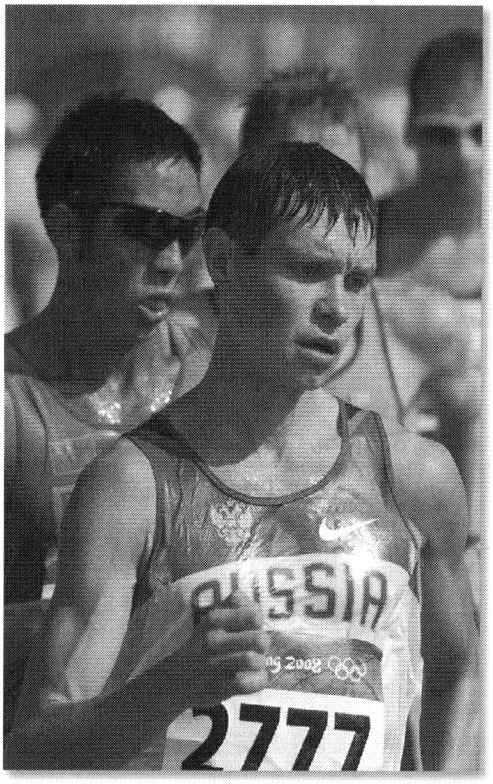

Denis Nizhegorodov - Russia
20km PR: 1:18:20, 50km PR: 3:34:14
Two Time World Cup Champion
Silver and Bronze Olympic Medalist
World Record Holder

Weekly Notes

MONDAY

TUESDAY

WEDNESDAY

THURSDAY

FRIDAY

SATURDAY

SUNDAY

MONDAY	Date:	Location:	2nd workout:	
W/U Distance :	W/U Time:			
Workout Type:			Total Daily Distance:	
C/D Distance:	C/D Time:			
TUESDAY	Date:	Location:	2nd workout:	
W/U Distance :	W/U Time:			
Workout Type:			Total Daily Distance:	
C/D Distance:	C/D Time:			
WEDNESDAY	Date:	Location:	2nd workout:	
W/U Distance :	W/U Time:			
Workout Type:			Total Daily Distance:	
C/D Distance:	C/D Time:			
THURSDAY	Date:	Location:	2nd workout:	
W/U Distance :	W/U Time:			
Workout Type:			Total Daily Distance:	
C/D Distance:	C/D Time:			
FRIDAY	Date:	Location:	2nd workout:	
W/U Distance :	W/U Time:			
Workout Type:			Total Daily Distance:	
C/D Distance:	C/D Time:			
SATURDAY	Date:	Location:	2nd workout:	
W/U Distance :	W/U Time:			
Workout Type:			Total Daily Distance:	
C/D Distance:	C/D Time:			
SUNDAY	Date:	Location:	2nd workout:	
W/U Distance :	W/U Time:			
Workout Type:			Total Daily Distance:	
C/D Distance:	C/D Time:			
		Total Distance for the Week:		

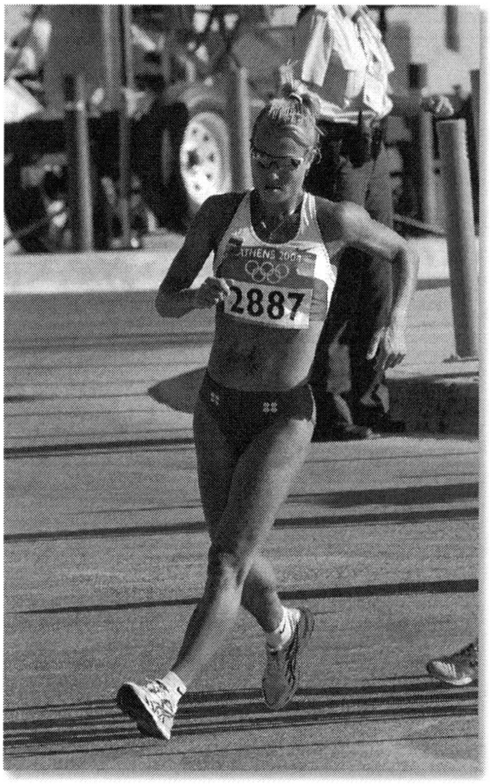

Olimpiada Ivanova – Russia
20km PR: 1:24:20
Three Time World Champion
Silver Medalist - Olympic Games
Silver Medalist - World Cup
World Record Holder

Weekly Notes

MONDAY

TUESDAY

WEDNESDAY

THURSDAY

FRIDAY

SATURDAY

SUNDAY

MONDAY	Date:	Location:	2nd workout:	
W/U Distance :		W/U Time:		
Workout Type:			Total Daily Distance:	
C/D Distance:		C/D Time:		

TUESDAY	Date:	Location:	2nd workout:	
W/U Distance :		W/U Time:		
Workout Type:			Total Daily Distance:	
C/D Distance:		C/D Time:		

WEDNESDAY	Date:	Location:	2nd workout:	
W/U Distance :		W/U Time:		
Workout Type:			Total Daily Distance:	
C/D Distance:		C/D Time:		

THURSDAY	Date:	Location:	2nd workout:	
W/U Distance :		W/U Time:		
Workout Type:			Total Daily Distance:	
C/D Distance:		C/D Time:		

FRIDAY	Date:	Location:	2nd workout:	
W/U Distance :		W/U Time:		
Workout Type:			Total Daily Distance:	
C/D Distance:		C/D Time:		

SATURDAY	Date:	Location:	2nd workout:	
W/U Distance :		W/U Time:		
Workout Type:			Total Daily Distance:	
C/D Distance:		C/D Time:		

SUNDAY	Date:	Location:	2nd workout:	
W/U Distance :		W/U Time:		
Workout Type:			Total Daily Distance:	
C/D Distance:		C/D Time:		

Total Distance for the Week:	

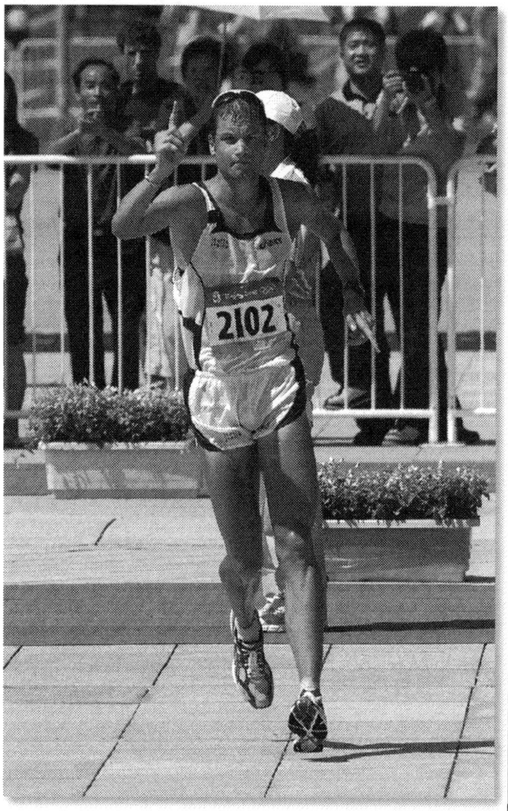

Alex Schwazer – Italy
20km PR: 1:21:38, 50km PR: 3:36:04
Olympic Champion, Two Time Bronze Medalist World Championships, Silver Medalist World Cup

Weekly Notes

MONDAY

TUESDAY

WEDNESDAY

THURSDAY

FRIDAY

SATURDAY

SUNDAY

MONDAY	Date:	Location:	2nd workout:	
W/U Distance :		W/U Time:		
Workout Type:			Total Daily Distance:	
C/D Distance:		C/D Time:		

TUESDAY	Date:	Location:	2nd workout:	
W/U Distance :		W/U Time:		
Workout Type:			Total Daily Distance:	
C/D Distance:		C/D Time:		

WEDNESDAY	Date:	Location:	2nd workout:	
W/U Distance :		W/U Time:		
Workout Type:			Total Daily Distance:	
C/D Distance:		C/D Time:		

THURSDAY	Date:	Location:	2nd workout:	
W/U Distance :		W/U Time:		
Workout Type:			Total Daily Distance:	
C/D Distance:		C/D Time:		

FRIDAY	Date:	Location:	2nd workout:	
W/U Distance :		W/U Time:		
Workout Type:			Total Daily Distance:	
C/D Distance:		C/D Time:		

SATURDAY	Date:	Location:	2nd workout:	
W/U Distance :		W/U Time:		
Workout Type:			Total Daily Distance:	
C/D Distance:		C/D Time:		

SUNDAY	Date:	Location:	2nd workout:	
W/U Distance :		W/U Time:		
Workout Type:			Total Daily Distance:	
C/D Distance:		C/D Time:		

Total Distance for the Week:	

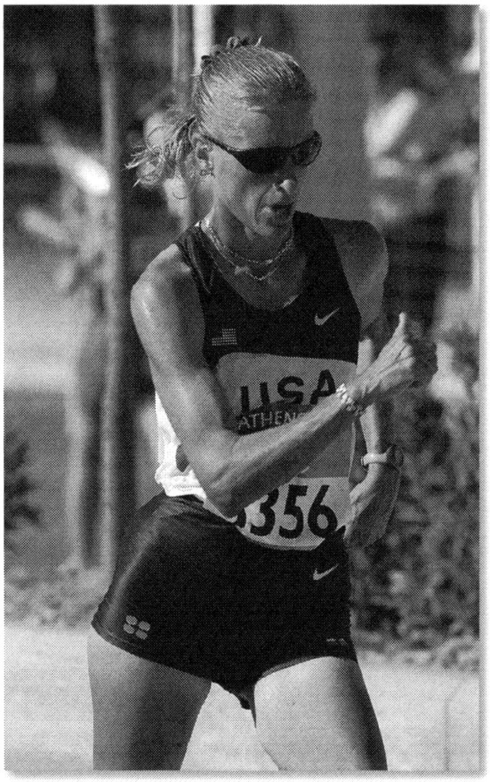

Teresa Vaill – USA
20km PR: 1:33:23
Olympian

Weekly Notes

MONDAY
TUESDAY
WEDNESDAY
THURSDAY
FRIDAY
SATURDAY
SUNDAY

MONDAY	Date:	Location:	2nd workout:	
W/U Distance :	W/U Time:			
Workout Type:			Total Daily Distance:	
C/D Distance:	C/D Time:			
TUESDAY	Date:	Location:	2nd workout:	
W/U Distance :	W/U Time:			
Workout Type:			Total Daily Distance:	
C/D Distance:	C/D Time:			
WEDNESDAY	Date:	Location:	2nd workout:	
W/U Distance :	W/U Time:			
Workout Type:			Total Daily Distance:	
C/D Distance:	C/D Time:			
THURSDAY	Date:	Location:	2nd workout:	
W/U Distance :	W/U Time:			
Workout Type:			Total Daily Distance:	
C/D Distance:	C/D Time:			
FRIDAY	Date:	Location:	2nd workout:	
W/U Distance :	W/U Time:			
Workout Type:			Total Daily Distance:	
C/D Distance:	C/D Time:			
SATURDAY	Date:	Location:	2nd workout:	
W/U Distance :	W/U Time:			
Workout Type:			Total Daily Distance:	
C/D Distance:	C/D Time:			
SUNDAY	Date:	Location:	2nd workout:	
W/U Distance :	W/U Time:			
Workout Type:			Total Daily Distance:	
C/D Distance:	C/D Time:			
		Total Distance for the Week:		

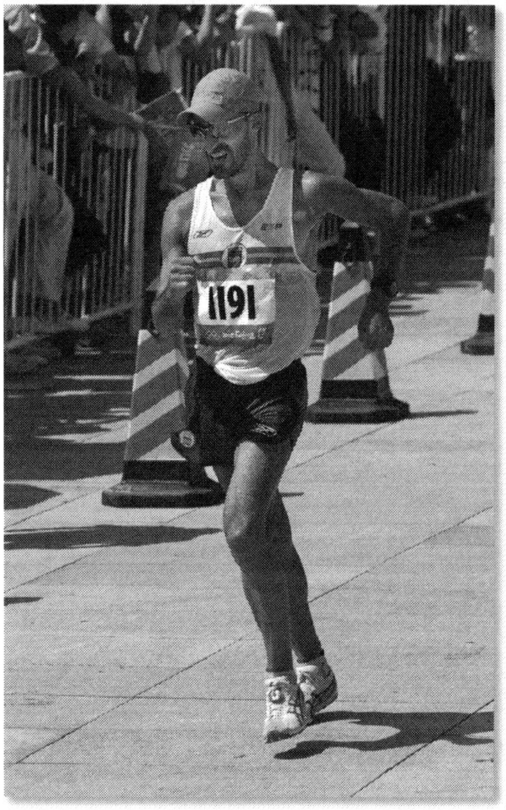

Jesús Angel García – Spain
20km PR: 1:23:00, 50km PR: 3:39:54
World Cup & World Champion

Weekly Notes

MONDAY

TUESDAY

WEDNESDAY

THURSDAY

FRIDAY

SATURDAY

SUNDAY

MONDAY	Date:	Location:	2nd workout:
W/U Distance :	W/U Time:		
Workout Type:			Total Daily Distance:
C/D Distance:	C/D Time:		

TUESDAY	Date:	Location:	2nd workout:
W/U Distance :	W/U Time:		
Workout Type:			Total Daily Distance:
C/D Distance:	C/D Time:		

WEDNESDAY	Date:	Location:	2nd workout:
W/U Distance :	W/U Time:		
Workout Type:			Total Daily Distance:
C/D Distance:	C/D Time:		

THURSDAY	Date:	Location:	2nd workout:
W/U Distance :	W/U Time:		
Workout Type:			Total Daily Distance:
C/D Distance:	C/D Time:		

FRIDAY	Date:	Location:	2nd workout:
W/U Distance :	W/U Time:		
Workout Type:			Total Daily Distance:
C/D Distance:	C/D Time:		

SATURDAY	Date:	Location:	2nd workout:
W/U Distance :	W/U Time:		
Workout Type:			Total Daily Distance:
C/D Distance:	C/D Time:		

SUNDAY	Date:	Location:	2nd workout:
W/U Distance :	W/U Time:		
Workout Type:			Total Daily Distance:
C/D Distance:	C/D Time:		

Total Distance for the Week:	

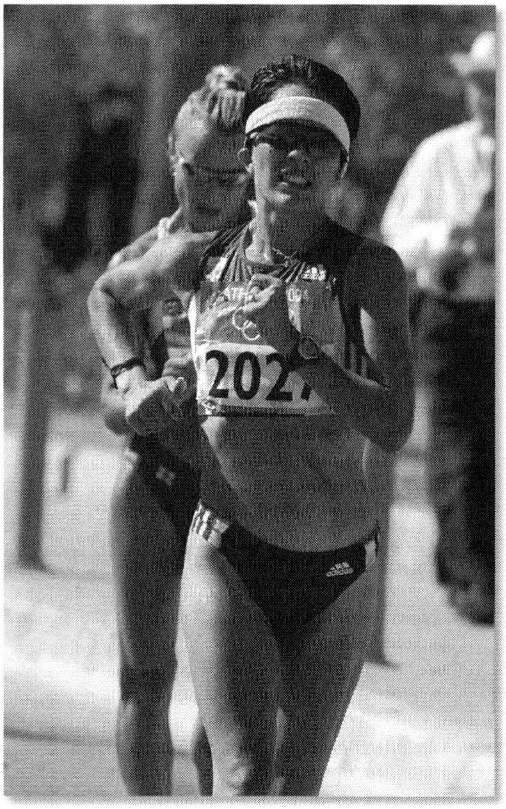

Anastasia Tsoumeléka - Greece
20km PR: 1:29:12
Olympic Champion

Weekly Notes

MONDAY
TUESDAY
WEDNESDAY
THURSDAY
FRIDAY
SATURDAY
SUNDAY

MONDAY	Date:	Location:	2nd workout:
W/U Distance :	W/U Time:		
Workout Type:			
C/D Distance:	C/D Time:	Total Daily Distance:	
TUESDAY	Date:	Location:	2nd workout:
W/U Distance :	W/U Time:		
Workout Type:			
C/D Distance:	C/D Time:	Total Daily Distance:	
WEDNESDAY	Date:	Location:	2nd workout:
W/U Distance :	W/U Time:		
Workout Type:			
C/D Distance:	C/D Time:	Total Daily Distance:	
THURSDAY	Date:	Location:	2nd workout:
W/U Distance :	W/U Time:		
Workout Type:			
C/D Distance:	C/D Time:	Total Daily Distance:	
FRIDAY	Date:	Location:	2nd workout:
W/U Distance :	W/U Time:		
Workout Type:			
C/D Distance:	C/D Time:	Total Daily Distance:	
SATURDAY	Date:	Location:	2nd workout:
W/U Distance :	W/U Time:		
Workout Type:			
C/D Distance:	C/D Time:	Total Daily Distance:	
SUNDAY	Date:	Location:	2nd workout:
W/U Distance :	W/U Time:		
Workout Type:			
C/D Distance:	C/D Time:	Total Daily Distance:	
		Total Distance for the Week:	

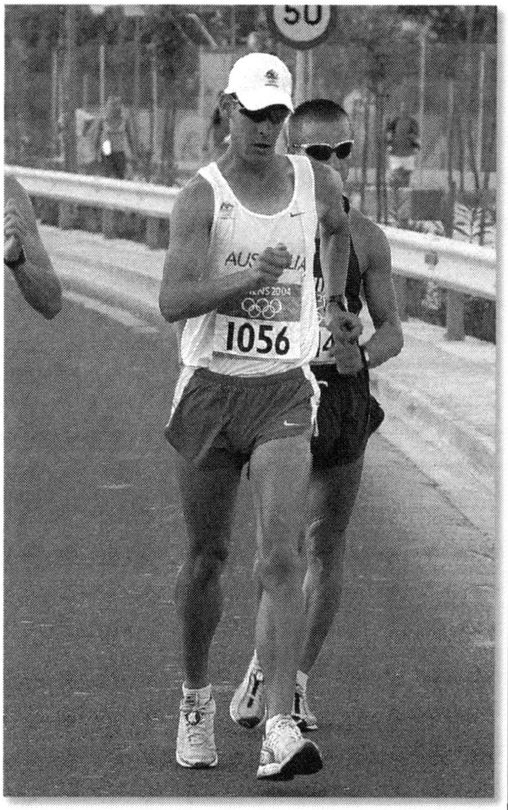

Nathan Deakes – Australia
20km PR: 1:17:33, 50km PR: 3:35:47
World Champion, Bronze Medalist – World Cup & Olympic Games
Former World Record Holder

Weekly Notes

MONDAY
TUESDAY
WEDNESDAY
THURSDAY
FRIDAY
SATURDAY
SUNDAY

MONDAY	Date:	Location:	2nd workout:	
W/U Distance :	W/U Time:			
Workout Type:				
C/D Distance:	C/D Time:		Total Daily Distance:	
TUESDAY	Date:	Location:	2nd workout:	
W/U Distance :	W/U Time:			
Workout Type:				
C/D Distance:	C/D Time:		Total Daily Distance:	
WEDNESDAY	Date:	Location:	2nd workout:	
W/U Distance :	W/U Time:			
Workout Type:				
C/D Distance:	C/D Time:		Total Daily Distance:	
THURSDAY	Date:	Location:	2nd workout:	
W/U Distance :	W/U Time:			
Workout Type:				
C/D Distance:	C/D Time:		Total Daily Distance:	
FRIDAY	Date:	Location:	2nd workout:	
W/U Distance :	W/U Time:			
Workout Type:				
C/D Distance:	C/D Time:		Total Daily Distance:	
SATURDAY	Date:	Location:	2nd workout:	
W/U Distance :	W/U Time:			
Workout Type:				
C/D Distance:	C/D Time:		Total Daily Distance:	
SUNDAY	Date:	Location:	2nd workout:	
W/U Distance :	W/U Time:			
Workout Type:				
C/D Distance:	C/D Time:		Total Daily Distance:	
		Total Distance for the Week:		

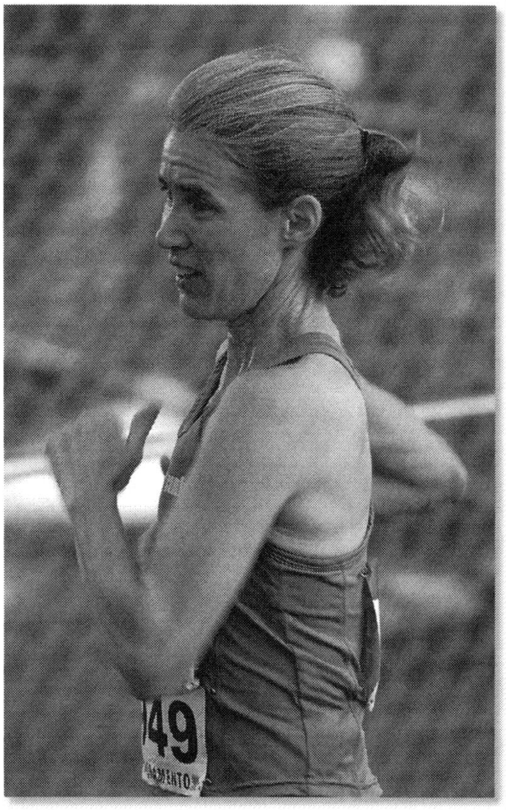

Michelle Rohl – USA
20km PR: 1:31:51
Three Time Olympian, US Record Holder

Weekly Notes

MONDAY

TUESDAY

WEDNESDAY

THURSDAY

FRIDAY

SATURDAY

SUNDAY

MONDAY	Date:	Location:	2nd workout:
W/U Distance :		W/U Time:	
Workout Type:			Total Daily Distance:
C/D Distance:		C/D Time:	

TUESDAY	Date:	Location:	2nd workout:
W/U Distance :		W/U Time:	
Workout Type:			Total Daily Distance:
C/D Distance:		C/D Time:	

WEDNESDAY	Date:	Location:	2nd workout:
W/U Distance :		W/U Time:	
Workout Type:			Total Daily Distance:
C/D Distance:		C/D Time:	

THURSDAY	Date:	Location:	2nd workout:
W/U Distance :		W/U Time:	
Workout Type:			Total Daily Distance:
C/D Distance:		C/D Time:	

FRIDAY	Date:	Location:	2nd workout:
W/U Distance :		W/U Time:	
Workout Type:			Total Daily Distance:
C/D Distance:		C/D Time:	

SATURDAY	Date:	Location:	2nd workout:
W/U Distance :		W/U Time:	
Workout Type:			Total Daily Distance:
C/D Distance:		C/D Time:	

SUNDAY	Date:	Location:	2nd workout:
W/U Distance :		W/U Time:	
Workout Type:			Total Daily Distance:
C/D Distance:		C/D Time:	

Total Distance for the Week:	

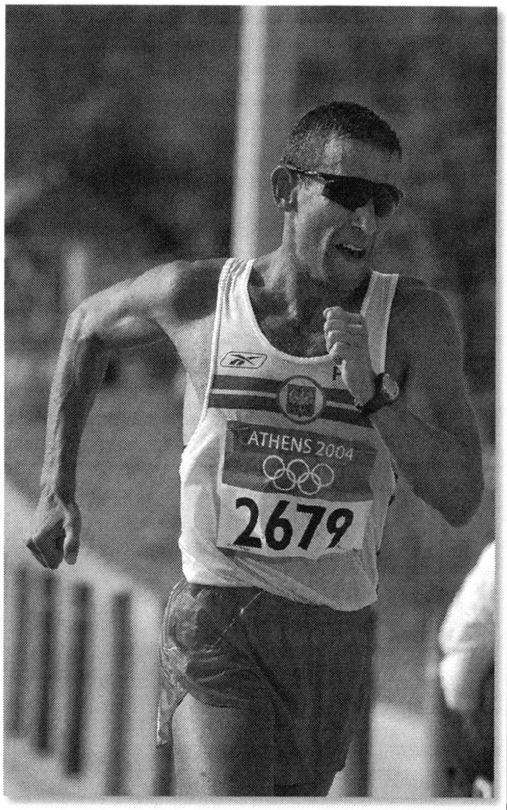

Robert Korzeniowski – Poland
20km PR: 1:18:22, 50km PR: 3:36.03
Four Time Olympic Gold Medalist
Three Time World Champion
Former World Record Holder

Weekly Notes

MONDAY

TUESDAY

WEDNESDAY

THURSDAY

FRIDAY

SATURDAY

SUNDAY

MONDAY	Date:	Location:	2nd workout:
W/U Distance :	W/U Time:		
Workout Type:			Total Daily Distance:
C/D Distance:	C/D Time:		

TUESDAY	Date:	Location:	2nd workout:
W/U Distance :	W/U Time:		
Workout Type:			Total Daily Distance:
C/D Distance:	C/D Time:		

WEDNESDAY	Date:	Location:	2nd workout:
W/U Distance :	W/U Time:		
Workout Type:			Total Daily Distance:
C/D Distance:	C/D Time:		

THURSDAY	Date:	Location:	2nd workout:
W/U Distance :	W/U Time:		
Workout Type:			Total Daily Distance:
C/D Distance:	C/D Time:		

FRIDAY	Date:	Location:	2nd workout:
W/U Distance :	W/U Time:		
Workout Type:			Total Daily Distance:
C/D Distance:	C/D Time:		

SATURDAY	Date:	Location:	2nd workout:
W/U Distance :	W/U Time:		
Workout Type:			Total Daily Distance:
C/D Distance:	C/D Time:		

SUNDAY	Date:	Location:	2nd workout:
W/U Distance :	W/U Time:		
Workout Type:			Total Daily Distance:
C/D Distance:	C/D Time:		

Total Distance for the Week:	

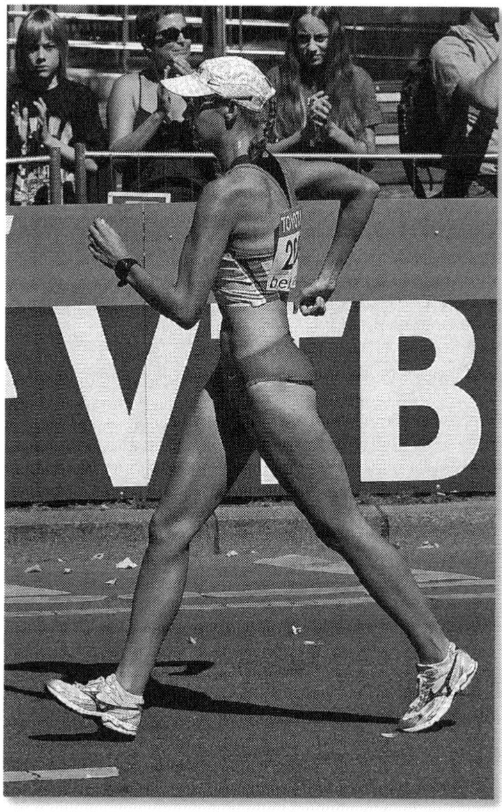

Rachel Lavallee – Canada
20km PR: 1:37:22
Canadian Jr. Record Holder
Olympic Hopeful

Weekly Notes

MONDAY

TUESDAY

WEDNESDAY

THURSDAY

FRIDAY

SATURDAY

SUNDAY

MONDAY	Date:	Location:	2nd workout:	
W/U Distance :		W/U Time:		
Workout Type:				
C/D Distance:		C/D Time:	Total Daily Distance:	

TUESDAY	Date:	Location:	2nd workout:	
W/U Distance :		W/U Time:		
Workout Type:				
C/D Distance:		C/D Time:	Total Daily Distance:	

WEDNESDAY	Date:	Location:	2nd workout:	
W/U Distance :		W/U Time:		
Workout Type:				
C/D Distance:		C/D Time:	Total Daily Distance:	

THURSDAY	Date:	Location:	2nd workout:	
W/U Distance :		W/U Time:		
Workout Type:				
C/D Distance:		C/D Time:	Total Daily Distance:	

FRIDAY	Date:	Location:	2nd workout:	
W/U Distance :		W/U Time:		
Workout Type:				
C/D Distance:		C/D Time:	Total Daily Distance:	

SATURDAY	Date:	Location:	2nd workout:	
W/U Distance :		W/U Time:		
Workout Type:				
C/D Distance:		C/D Time:	Total Daily Distance:	

SUNDAY	Date:	Location:	2nd workout:	
W/U Distance :		W/U Time:		
Workout Type:				
C/D Distance:		C/D Time:	Total Daily Distance:	

Total Distance for the Week:	

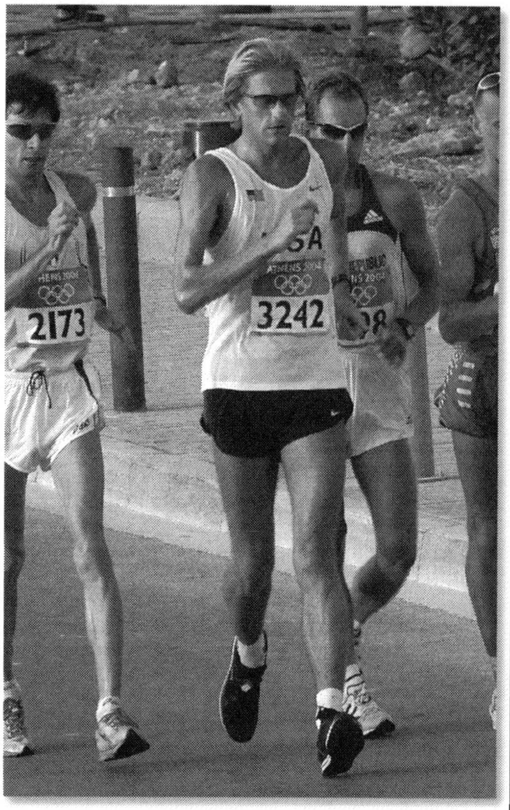

Curt Clausen – USA
20km PR: 1:23:34, 50km PR: 3:48:04
29 time US National Champion
US 50km Record Holder
Bronze Medalist -World Championships

Weekly Notes

MONDAY

TUESDAY

WEDNESDAY

THURSDAY

FRIDAY

SATURDAY

SUNDAY

MONDAY	Date:	Location:	2nd workout:	
W/U Distance :	W/U Time:			
Workout Type:			Total Daily Distance:	
C/D Distance:	C/D Time:			

TUESDAY	Date:	Location:	2nd workout:	
W/U Distance :	W/U Time:			
Workout Type:			Total Daily Distance:	
C/D Distance:	C/D Time:			

WEDNESDAY	Date:	Location:	2nd workout:	
W/U Distance :	W/U Time:			
Workout Type:			Total Daily Distance:	
C/D Distance:	C/D Time:			

THURSDAY	Date:	Location:	2nd workout:	
W/U Distance :	W/U Time:			
Workout Type:			Total Daily Distance:	
C/D Distance:	C/D Time:			

FRIDAY	Date:	Location:	2nd workout:	
W/U Distance :	W/U Time:			
Workout Type:			Total Daily Distance:	
C/D Distance:	C/D Time:			

SATURDAY	Date:	Location:	2nd workout:	
W/U Distance :	W/U Time:			
Workout Type:			Total Daily Distance:	
C/D Distance:	C/D Time:			

SUNDAY	Date:	Location:	2nd workout:	
W/U Distance :	W/U Time:			
Workout Type:			Total Daily Distance:	
C/D Distance:	C/D Time:			

Total Distance for the Week:	

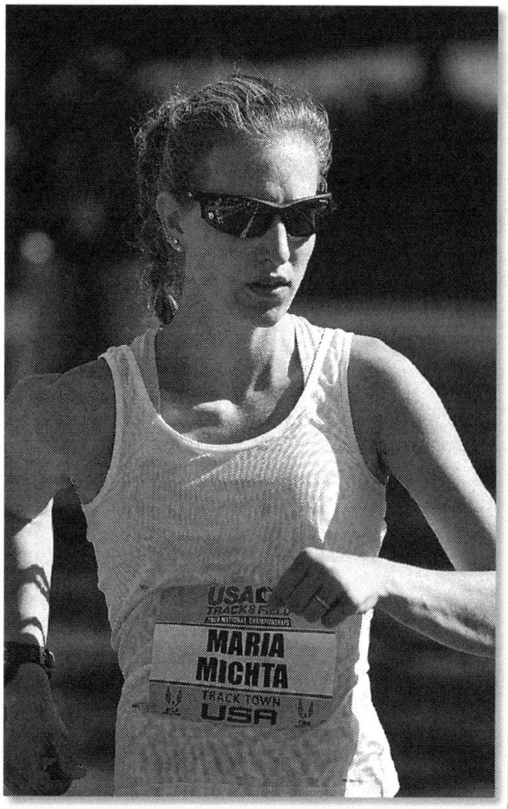

Maria Michta – USA
20km PR: 1:41:16
US Junior Record Holder, Olympic Hopeful

Weekly Notes

MONDAY

TUESDAY

WEDNESDAY

THURSDAY

FRIDAY

SATURDAY

SUNDAY

MONDAY	Date:	Location:	2nd workout:	
W/U Distance :		W/U Time:		
Workout Type:			Total Daily Distance:	
C/D Distance:		C/D Time:		

TUESDAY	Date:	Location:	2nd workout:	
W/U Distance :		W/U Time:		
Workout Type:			Total Daily Distance:	
C/D Distance:		C/D Time:		

WEDNESDAY	Date:	Location:	2nd workout:	
W/U Distance :		W/U Time:		
Workout Type:			Total Daily Distance:	
C/D Distance:		C/D Time:		

THURSDAY	Date:	Location:	2nd workout:	
W/U Distance :		W/U Time:		
Workout Type:			Total Daily Distance:	
C/D Distance:		C/D Time:		

FRIDAY	Date:	Location:	2nd workout:	
W/U Distance :		W/U Time:		
Workout Type:			Total Daily Distance:	
C/D Distance:		C/D Time:		

SATURDAY	Date:	Location:	2nd workout:	
W/U Distance :		W/U Time:		
Workout Type:			Total Daily Distance:	
C/D Distance:		C/D Time:		

SUNDAY	Date:	Location:	2nd workout:	
W/U Distance :		W/U Time:		
Workout Type:			Total Daily Distance:	
C/D Distance:		C/D Time:		

Total Distance for the Week:	

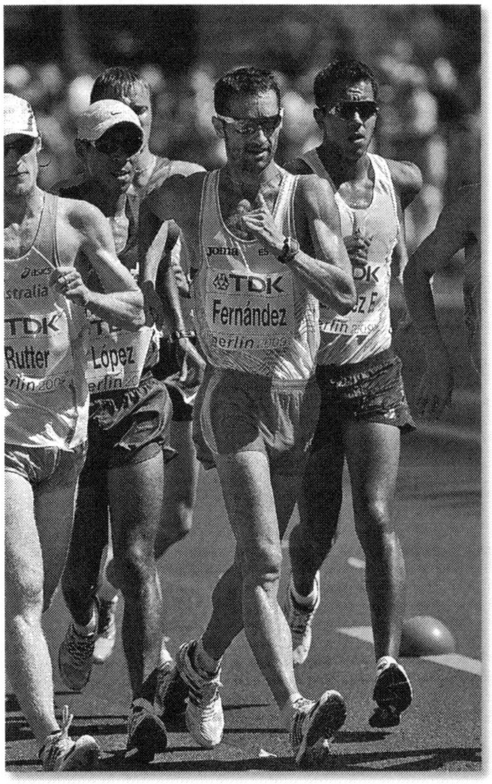

Francisco Javier Fernández - Spain
Two time World Cup Champion
Silver Medalist – Olympic Games
20km PR: 1:17:22, 50km PR: 3:41:02

Weekly Notes

MONDAY

TUESDAY

WEDNESDAY

THURSDAY

FRIDAY

SATURDAY

SUNDAY

MONDAY	**Date:**	**Location:**	**2nd workout:**
W/U Distance :		**W/U Time:**	
Workout Type:			**Total Daily Distance:**
C/D Distance:		**C/D Time:**	
TUESDAY	**Date:**	**Location:**	**2nd workout:**
W/U Distance :		**W/U Time:**	
Workout Type:			**Total Daily Distance:**
C/D Distance:		**C/D Time:**	
WEDNESDAY	**Date:**	**Location:**	**2nd workout:**
W/U Distance :		**W/U Time:**	
Workout Type:			**Total Daily Distance:**
C/D Distance:		**C/D Time:**	
THURSDAY	**Date:**	**Location:**	**2nd workout:**
W/U Distance :		**W/U Time:**	
Workout Type:			**Total Daily Distance:**
C/D Distance:		**C/D Time:**	
FRIDAY	**Date:**	**Location:**	**2nd workout:**
W/U Distance :		**W/U Time:**	
Workout Type:			**Total Daily Distance:**
C/D Distance:		**C/D Time:**	
SATURDAY	**Date:**	**Location:**	**2nd workout:**
W/U Distance :		**W/U Time:**	
Workout Type:			**Total Daily Distance:**
C/D Distance:		**C/D Time:**	
SUNDAY	**Date:**	**Location:**	**2nd workout:**
W/U Distance :		**W/U Time:**	
Workout Type:			**Total Daily Distance:**
C/D Distance:		**C/D Time:**	
		Total Distance for the Week:	

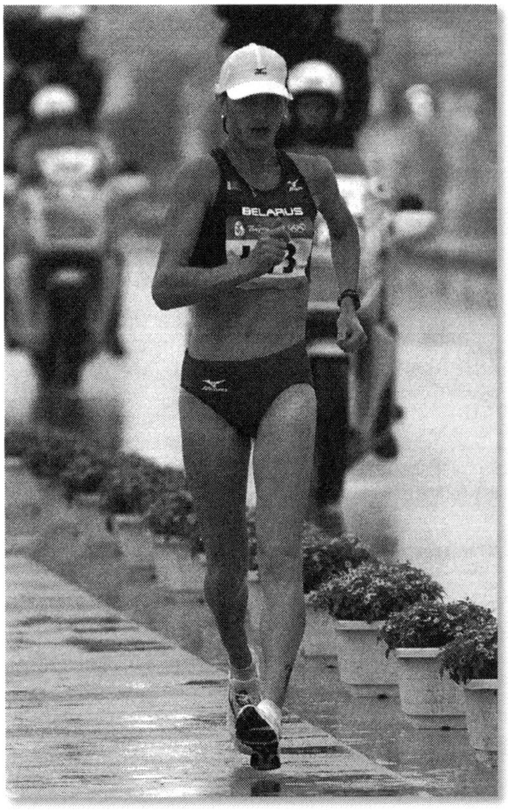

Rita Turava – Belarus
20km PR: 1:26:11
Silver Medalist – World Cup

Weekly Notes

MONDAY

TUESDAY

WEDNESDAY

THURSDAY

FRIDAY

SATURDAY

SUNDAY

MONDAY	Date:	Location:	2nd workout:
W/U Distance :	W/U Time:		
Workout Type:			Total Daily Distance:
C/D Distance:	C/D Time:		
TUESDAY	Date:	Location:	2nd workout:
W/U Distance :	W/U Time:		
Workout Type:			Total Daily Distance:
C/D Distance:	C/D Time:		
WEDNESDAY	Date:	Location:	2nd workout:
W/U Distance :	W/U Time:		
Workout Type:			Total Daily Distance:
C/D Distance:	C/D Time:		
THURSDAY	Date:	Location:	2nd workout:
W/U Distance :	W/U Time:		
Workout Type:			Total Daily Distance:
C/D Distance:	C/D Time:		
FRIDAY	Date:	Location:	2nd workout:
W/U Distance :	W/U Time:		
Workout Type:			Total Daily Distance:
C/D Distance:	C/D Time:		
SATURDAY	Date:	Location:	2nd workout:
W/U Distance :	W/U Time:		
Workout Type:			Total Daily Distance:
C/D Distance:	C/D Time:		
SUNDAY	Date:	Location:	2nd workout:
W/U Distance :	W/U Time:		
Workout Type:			Total Daily Distance:
C/D Distance:	C/D Time:		
		Total Distance for the Week:	

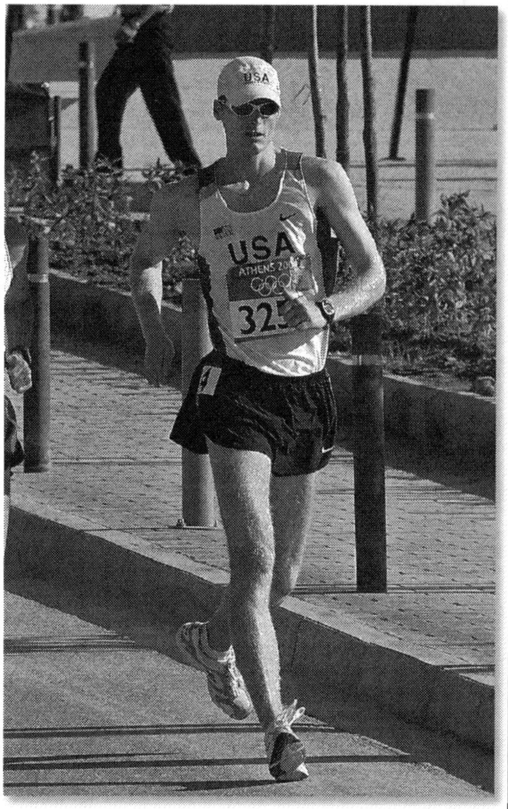

Kevin Eastler – USA
20km PR: 1:22:25, 50km PR: 4:05:44
Two Time Olympian
US 30km Record Holder

Weekly Notes

MONDAY

TUESDAY

WEDNESDAY

THURSDAY

FRIDAY

SATURDAY

SUNDAY

MONDAY	Date:	Location:	2nd workout:	
W/U Distance :		W/U Time:		
Workout Type:			Total Daily Distance:	
C/D Distance:		C/D Time:		

TUESDAY	Date:	Location:	2nd workout:	
W/U Distance :		W/U Time:		
Workout Type:			Total Daily Distance:	
C/D Distance:		C/D Time:		

WEDNESDAY	Date:	Location:	2nd workout:	
W/U Distance :		W/U Time:		
Workout Type:			Total Daily Distance:	
C/D Distance:		C/D Time:		

THURSDAY	Date:	Location:	2nd workout:	
W/U Distance :		W/U Time:		
Workout Type:			Total Daily Distance:	
C/D Distance:		C/D Time:		

FRIDAY	Date:	Location:	2nd workout:	
W/U Distance :		W/U Time:		
Workout Type:			Total Daily Distance:	
C/D Distance:		C/D Time:		

SATURDAY	Date:	Location:	2nd workout:	
W/U Distance :		W/U Time:		
Workout Type:			Total Daily Distance:	
C/D Distance:		C/D Time:		

SUNDAY	Date:	Location:	2nd workout:	
W/U Distance :		W/U Time:		
Workout Type:			Total Daily Distance:	
C/D Distance:		C/D Time:		

Total Distance for the Week:	

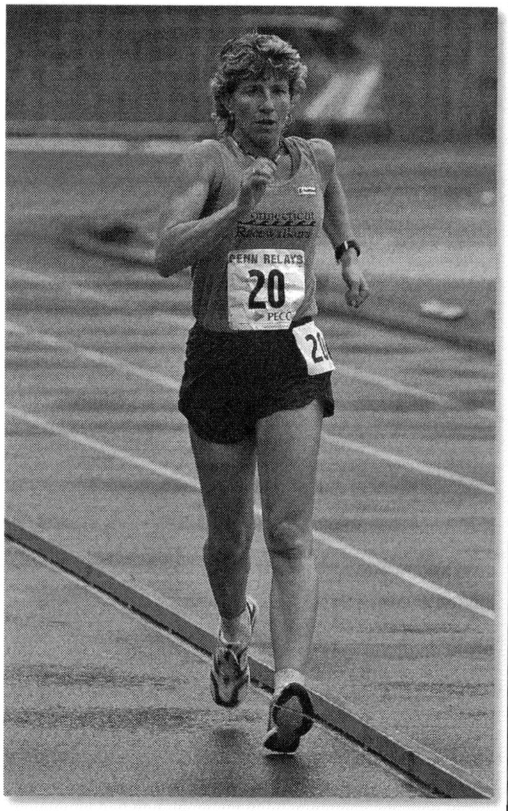

Maryanne Daniel
10km PR: 46:17
Six Time National Champion

Weekly Notes

MONDAY

TUESDAY

WEDNESDAY

THURSDAY

FRIDAY

SATURDAY

SUNDAY

MONDAY	Date:	Location:	2nd workout:
W/U Distance :		W/U Time:	
Workout Type:			Total Daily Distance:
C/D Distance:		C/D Time:	
TUESDAY	Date:	Location:	2nd workout:
W/U Distance :		W/U Time:	
Workout Type:			Total Daily Distance:
C/D Distance:		C/D Time:	
WEDNESDAY	Date:	Location:	2nd workout:
W/U Distance :		W/U Time:	
Workout Type:			Total Daily Distance:
C/D Distance:		C/D Time:	
THURSDAY	Date:	Location:	2nd workout:
W/U Distance :		W/U Time:	
Workout Type:			Total Daily Distance:
C/D Distance:		C/D Time:	
FRIDAY	Date:	Location:	2nd workout:
W/U Distance :		W/U Time:	
Workout Type:			Total Daily Distance:
C/D Distance:		C/D Time:	
SATURDAY	Date:	Location:	2nd workout:
W/U Distance :		W/U Time:	
Workout Type:			Total Daily Distance:
C/D Distance:		C/D Time:	
SUNDAY	Date:	Location:	2nd workout:
W/U Distance :		W/U Time:	
Workout Type:			Total Daily Distance:
C/D Distance:		C/D Time:	
		Total Distance for the Week:	

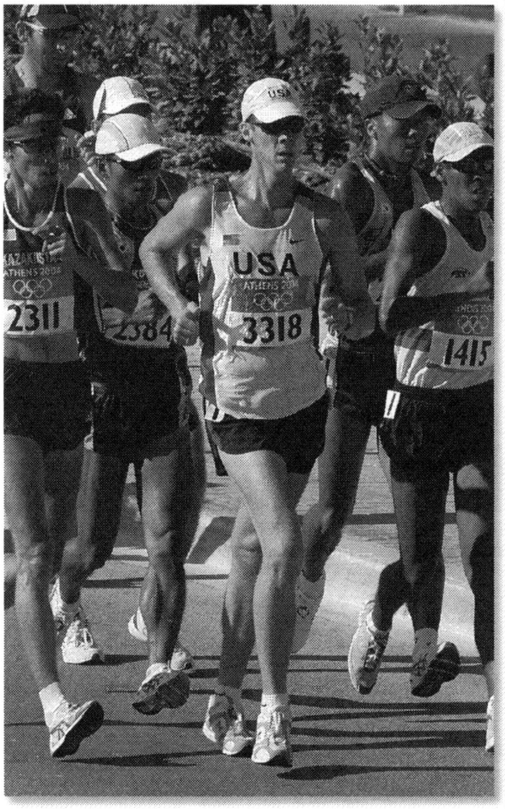

John Nunn – USA
20km PR: 1:22:31, 50km PR: 4:14:16
Olympian

Weekly Notes

MONDAY
TUESDAY
WEDNESDAY
THURSDAY
FRIDAY
SATURDAY
SUNDAY

MONDAY	Date:	Location:	2nd workout:	
W/U Distance :		W/U Time:		
Workout Type:				
			Total Daily Distance:	
C/D Distance:		C/D Time:		

TUESDAY	Date:	Location:	2nd workout:	
W/U Distance :		W/U Time:		
Workout Type:				
			Total Daily Distance:	
C/D Distance:		C/D Time:		

WEDNESDAY	Date:	Location:	2nd workout:	
W/U Distance :		W/U Time:		
Workout Type:				
			Total Daily Distance:	
C/D Distance:		C/D Time:		

THURSDAY	Date:	Location:	2nd workout:	
W/U Distance :		W/U Time:		
Workout Type:				
			Total Daily Distance:	
C/D Distance:		C/D Time:		

FRIDAY	Date:	Location:	2nd workout:	
W/U Distance :		W/U Time:		
Workout Type:				
			Total Daily Distance:	
C/D Distance:		C/D Time:		

SATURDAY	Date:	Location:	2nd workout:	
W/U Distance :		W/U Time:		
Workout Type:				
			Total Daily Distance:	
C/D Distance:		C/D Time:		

SUNDAY	Date:	Location:	2nd workout:	
W/U Distance :		W/U Time:		
Workout Type:				
			Total Daily Distance:	
C/D Distance:		C/D Time:		

Total Distance for the Week:	

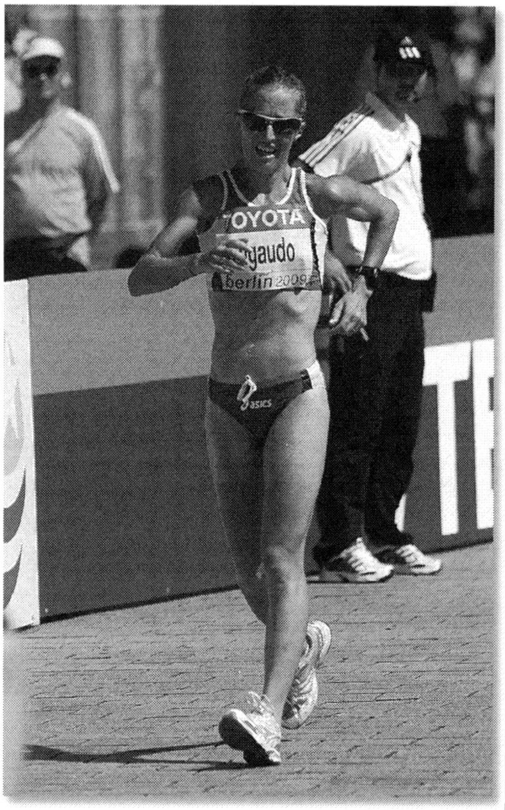

Elisa Rigaudo – Italy
20km PR: 1:27:12
Olympic Bronze Medalist

Weekly Notes

MONDAY

TUESDAY

WEDNESDAY

THURSDAY

FRIDAY

SATURDAY

SUNDAY

MONDAY	Date:	Location:	2nd workout:	
W/U Distance :	W/U Time:			
Workout Type:			Total Daily Distance:	
C/D Distance:	C/D Time:			

TUESDAY	Date:	Location:	2nd workout:	
W/U Distance :	W/U Time:			
Workout Type:			Total Daily Distance:	
C/D Distance:	C/D Time:			

WEDNESDAY	Date:	Location:	2nd workout:	
W/U Distance :	W/U Time:			
Workout Type:			Total Daily Distance:	
C/D Distance:	C/D Time:			

THURSDAY	Date:	Location:	2nd workout:	
W/U Distance :	W/U Time:			
Workout Type:			Total Daily Distance:	
C/D Distance:	C/D Time:			

FRIDAY	Date:	Location:	2nd workout:	
W/U Distance :	W/U Time:			
Workout Type:			Total Daily Distance:	
C/D Distance:	C/D Time:			

SATURDAY	Date:	Location:	2nd workout:	
W/U Distance :	W/U Time:			
Workout Type:			Total Daily Distance:	
C/D Distance:	C/D Time:			

SUNDAY	Date:	Location:	2nd workout:	
W/U Distance :	W/U Time:			
Workout Type:			Total Daily Distance:	
C/D Distance:	C/D Time:			

Total Distance for the Week:	

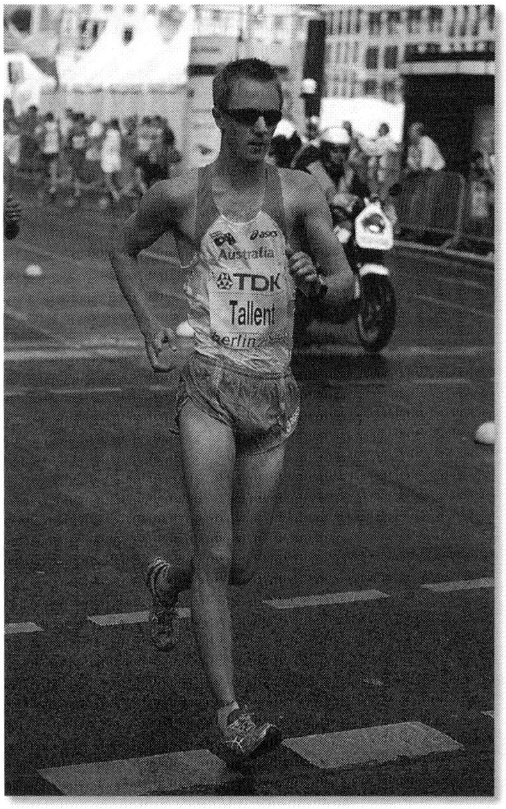

Jared Tallent – Australia
20km PR: 1:19:41 , 50km PR: 3:39:27
Olympic Silver and Bronze Medalist

Weekly Notes

MONDAY

TUESDAY

WEDNESDAY

THURSDAY

FRIDAY

SATURDAY

SUNDAY

MONDAY	Date:	Location:	2nd workout:
W/U Distance :		W/U Time:	
Workout Type:			
C/D Distance:		C/D Time:	Total Daily Distance:

TUESDAY	Date:	Location:	2nd workout:
W/U Distance :		W/U Time:	
Workout Type:			
C/D Distance:		C/D Time:	Total Daily Distance:

WEDNESDAY	Date:	Location:	2nd workout:
W/U Distance :		W/U Time:	
Workout Type:			
C/D Distance:		C/D Time:	Total Daily Distance:

THURSDAY	Date:	Location:	2nd workout:
W/U Distance :		W/U Time:	
Workout Type:			
C/D Distance:		C/D Time:	Total Daily Distance:

FRIDAY	Date:	Location:	2nd workout:
W/U Distance :		W/U Time:	
Workout Type:			
C/D Distance:		C/D Time:	Total Daily Distance:

SATURDAY	Date:	Location:	2nd workout:
W/U Distance :		W/U Time:	
Workout Type:			
C/D Distance:		C/D Time:	Total Daily Distance:

SUNDAY	Date:	Location:	2nd workout:
W/U Distance :		W/U Time:	
Workout Type:			
C/D Distance:		C/D Time:	Total Daily Distance:

Total Distance for the Week:	

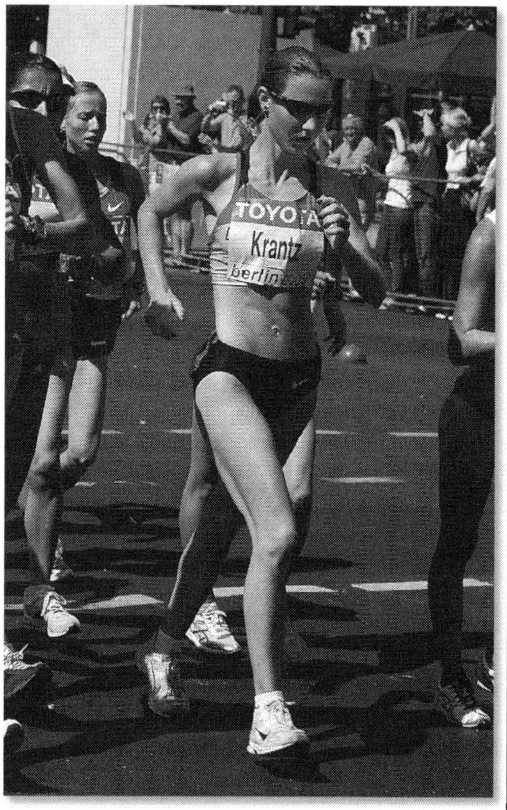

Sabine Krantz – Germany
20km PR: 1:27:56
World Junior Champion

Weekly Notes

MONDAY

TUESDAY

WEDNESDAY

THURSDAY

FRIDAY

SATURDAY

SUNDAY

MONDAY	Date:	Location:	2nd workout:
W/U Distance :		W/U Time:	
Workout Type:			Total Daily Distance:
C/D Distance:		C/D Time:	

TUESDAY	Date:	Location:	2nd workout:
W/U Distance :		W/U Time:	
Workout Type:			Total Daily Distance:
C/D Distance:		C/D Time:	

WEDNESDAY	Date:	Location:	2nd workout:
W/U Distance :		W/U Time:	
Workout Type:			Total Daily Distance:
C/D Distance:		C/D Time:	

THURSDAY	Date:	Location:	2nd workout:
W/U Distance :		W/U Time:	
Workout Type:			Total Daily Distance:
C/D Distance:		C/D Time:	

FRIDAY	Date:	Location:	2nd workout:
W/U Distance :		W/U Time:	
Workout Type:			Total Daily Distance:
C/D Distance:		C/D Time:	

SATURDAY	Date:	Location:	2nd workout:
W/U Distance :		W/U Time:	
Workout Type:			Total Daily Distance:
C/D Distance:		C/D Time:	

SUNDAY	Date:	Location:	2nd workout:
W/U Distance :		W/U Time:	
Workout Type:			Total Daily Distance:
C/D Distance:		C/D Time:	

Total Distance for the Week:	

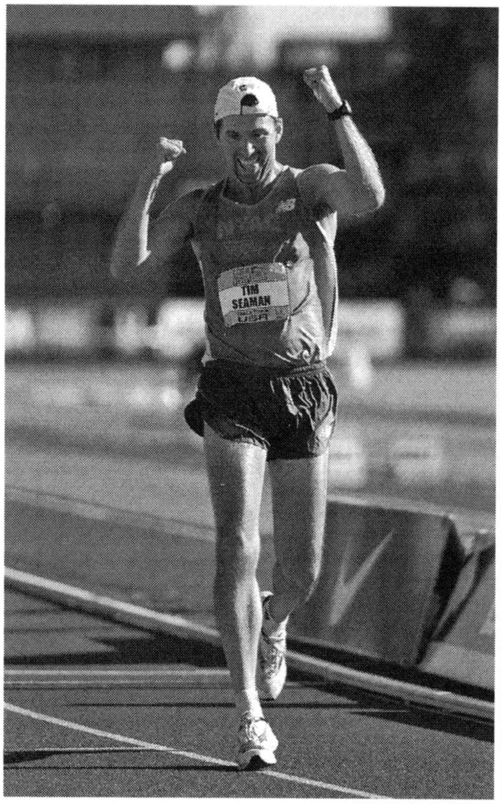

Tim Seaman – USA
20km PR: 1:22:02, 50km PR: 4:05:35
Two Time Olympian
US 20km Record Holder
38 Time National Champion

Weekly Notes

MONDAY

TUESDAY

WEDNESDAY

THURSDAY

FRIDAY

SATURDAY

SUNDAY

MONDAY	Date:	Location:	2nd workout:
W/U Distance :	W/U Time:		
Workout Type:			Total Daily Distance:
C/D Distance:	C/D Time:		

TUESDAY	Date:	Location:	2nd workout:
W/U Distance :	W/U Time:		
Workout Type:			Total Daily Distance:
C/D Distance:	C/D Time:		

WEDNESDAY	Date:	Location:	2nd workout:
W/U Distance :	W/U Time:		
Workout Type:			Total Daily Distance:
C/D Distance:	C/D Time:		

THURSDAY	Date:	Location:	2nd workout:
W/U Distance :	W/U Time:		
Workout Type:			Total Daily Distance:
C/D Distance:	C/D Time:		

FRIDAY	Date:	Location:	2nd workout:
W/U Distance :	W/U Time:		
Workout Type:			Total Daily Distance:
C/D Distance:	C/D Time:		

SATURDAY	Date:	Location:	2nd workout:
W/U Distance :	W/U Time:		
Workout Type:			Total Daily Distance:
C/D Distance:	C/D Time:		

SUNDAY	Date:	Location:	2nd workout:
W/U Distance :	W/U Time:		
Workout Type:			Total Daily Distance:
C/D Distance:	C/D Time:		

Total Distance for the Week:	

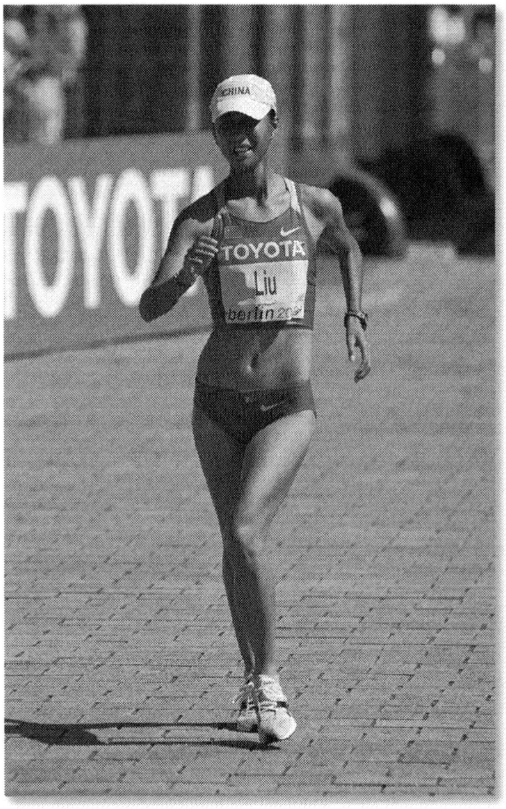

Hong Liu – China
20km PR: 1:27:17
World Championships Bronze Medalist

Weekly Notes

MONDAY
TUESDAY
WEDNESDAY
THURSDAY
FRIDAY
SATURDAY
SUNDAY

MONDAY	Date:	Location:	2nd workout:
W/U Distance :	W/U Time:		
Workout Type:			Total Daily Distance:
C/D Distance:	C/D Time:		

TUESDAY	Date:	Location:	2nd workout:
W/U Distance :	W/U Time:		
Workout Type:			Total Daily Distance:
C/D Distance:	C/D Time:		

WEDNESDAY	Date:	Location:	2nd workout:
W/U Distance :	W/U Time:		
Workout Type:			Total Daily Distance:
C/D Distance:	C/D Time:		

THURSDAY	Date:	Location:	2nd workout:
W/U Distance :	W/U Time:		
Workout Type:			Total Daily Distance:
C/D Distance:	C/D Time:		

FRIDAY	Date:	Location:	2nd workout:
W/U Distance :	W/U Time:		
Workout Type:			Total Daily Distance:
C/D Distance:	C/D Time:		

SATURDAY	Date:	Location:	2nd workout:
W/U Distance :	W/U Time:		
Workout Type:			Total Daily Distance:
C/D Distance:	C/D Time:		

SUNDAY	Date:	Location:	2nd workout:
W/U Distance :	W/U Time:		
Workout Type:			Total Daily Distance:
C/D Distance:	C/D Time:		

Total Distance for the Week:	

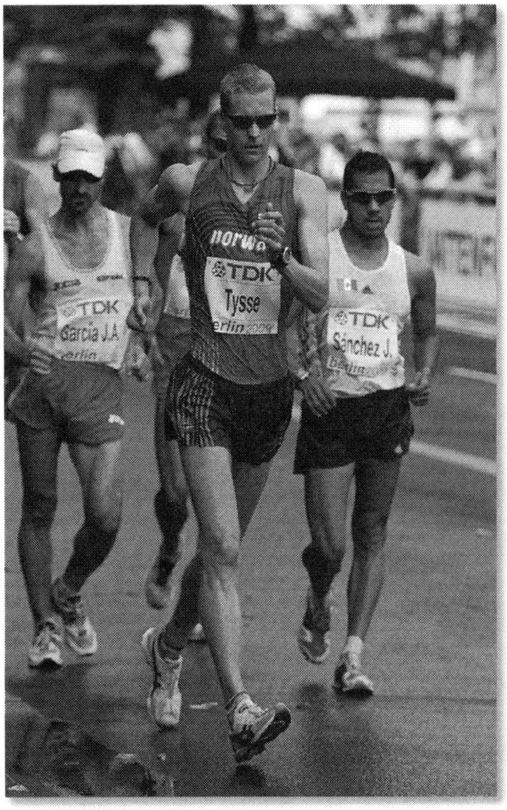

Erik "The Rocket" Tysse – Norway
20km PR: 1:19:11, 50km PR: 3:45:08
Two Time Olympian

Weekly Notes

MONDAY

TUESDAY

WEDNESDAY

THURSDAY

FRIDAY

SATURDAY

SUNDAY

MONDAY	Date:	Location:	2nd workout:	
W/U Distance :		W/U Time:		
Workout Type:			Total Daily Distance:	
C/D Distance:		C/D Time:		

TUESDAY	Date:	Location:	2nd workout:	
W/U Distance :		W/U Time:		
Workout Type:			Total Daily Distance:	
C/D Distance:		C/D Time:		

WEDNESDAY	Date:	Location:	2nd workout:	
W/U Distance :		W/U Time:		
Workout Type:			Total Daily Distance:	
C/D Distance:		C/D Time:		

THURSDAY	Date:	Location:	2nd workout:	
W/U Distance :		W/U Time:		
Workout Type:			Total Daily Distance:	
C/D Distance:		C/D Time:		

FRIDAY	Date:	Location:	2nd workout:	
W/U Distance :		W/U Time:		
Workout Type:			Total Daily Distance:	
C/D Distance:		C/D Time:		

SATURDAY	Date:	Location:	2nd workout:	
W/U Distance :		W/U Time:		
Workout Type:			Total Daily Distance:	
C/D Distance:		C/D Time:		

SUNDAY	Date:	Location:	2nd workout:	
W/U Distance :		W/U Time:		
Workout Type:			Total Daily Distance:	
C/D Distance:		C/D Time:		

Total Distance for the Week:	

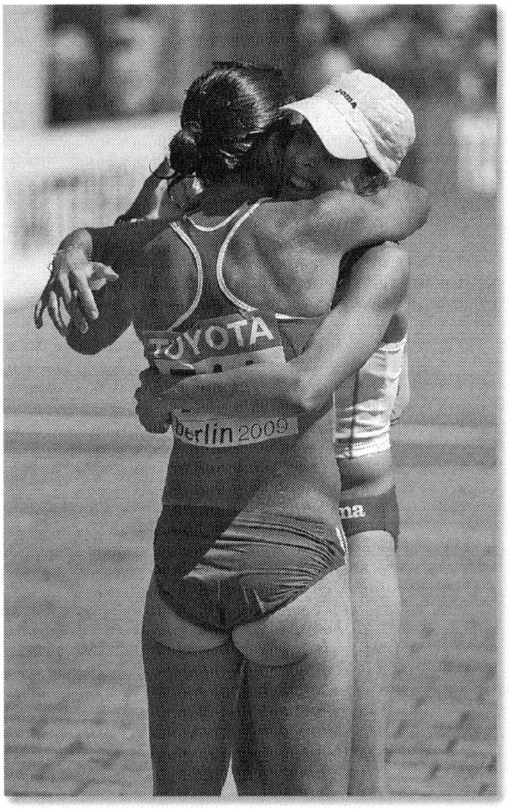

Vera Santos (Portugal) and Beatriz Pasqual (Spain) congratulating each other after finishing the World Championships

Weekly Notes

MONDAY

TUESDAY

WEDNESDAY

THURSDAY

FRIDAY

SATURDAY

SUNDAY

MONDAY	**Date:**	**Location:**	**2nd workout:**	
W/U Distance :	**W/U Time:**			
Workout Type:			**Total Daily Distance:**	
C/D Distance:	**C/D Time:**			
TUESDAY	**Date:**	**Location:**	**2nd workout:**	
W/U Distance :	**W/U Time:**			
Workout Type:			**Total Daily Distance:**	
C/D Distance:	**C/D Time:**			
WEDNESDAY	**Date:**	**Location:**	**2nd workout:**	
W/U Distance :	**W/U Time:**			
Workout Type:			**Total Daily Distance:**	
C/D Distance:	**C/D Time:**			
THURSDAY	**Date:**	**Location:**	**2nd workout:**	
W/U Distance :	**W/U Time:**			
Workout Type:			**Total Daily Distance:**	
C/D Distance:	**C/D Time:**			
FRIDAY	**Date:**	**Location:**	**2nd workout:**	
W/U Distance :	**W/U Time:**			
Workout Type:			**Total Daily Distance:**	
C/D Distance:	**C/D Time:**			
SATURDAY	**Date:**	**Location:**	**2nd workout:**	
W/U Distance :	**W/U Time:**			
Workout Type:			**Total Daily Distance:**	
C/D Distance:	**C/D Time:**			
SUNDAY	**Date:**	**Location:**	**2nd workout:**	
W/U Distance :	**W/U Time:**			
Workout Type:			**Total Daily Distance:**	
C/D Distance:	**C/D Time:**			
		Total Distance for the Week:		

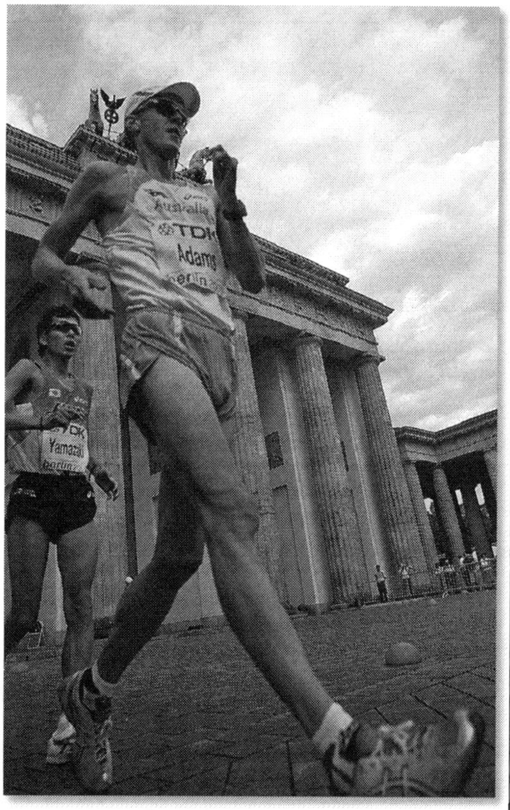

Luke Adams – Australia
20km PR: 1:19:15, 50km PR: 3:43:39
Three Time Commonwealth
Games Silver Medalist, Two Time IAAF
Race Walk Challenge Champion

Weekly Notes

MONDAY

TUESDAY

WEDNESDAY

THURSDAY

FRIDAY

SATURDAY

SUNDAY

MONDAY	**Date:**	**Location:**	**2nd workout:**
W/U Distance :	**W/U Time:**		
Workout Type:			**Total Daily Distance:**
C/D Distance:	**C/D Time:**		
TUESDAY	**Date:**	**Location:**	**2nd workout:**
W/U Distance :	**W/U Time:**		
Workout Type:			**Total Daily Distance:**
C/D Distance:	**C/D Time:**		
WEDNESDAY	**Date:**	**Location:**	**2nd workout:**
W/U Distance :	**W/U Time:**		
Workout Type:			**Total Daily Distance:**
C/D Distance:	**C/D Time:**		
THURSDAY	**Date:**	**Location:**	**2nd workout:**
W/U Distance :	**W/U Time:**		
Workout Type:			**Total Daily Distance:**
C/D Distance:	**C/D Time:**		
FRIDAY	**Date:**	**Location:**	**2nd workout:**
W/U Distance :	**W/U Time:**		
Workout Type:			**Total Daily Distance:**
C/D Distance:	**C/D Time:**		
SATURDAY	**Date:**	**Location:**	**2nd workout:**
W/U Distance :	**W/U Time:**		
Workout Type:			**Total Daily Distance:**
C/D Distance:	**C/D Time:**		
SUNDAY	**Date:**	**Location:**	**2nd workout:**
W/U Distance :	**W/U Time:**		
Workout Type:			**Total Daily Distance:**
C/D Distance:	**C/D Time:**		
		Total Distance for the Week:	

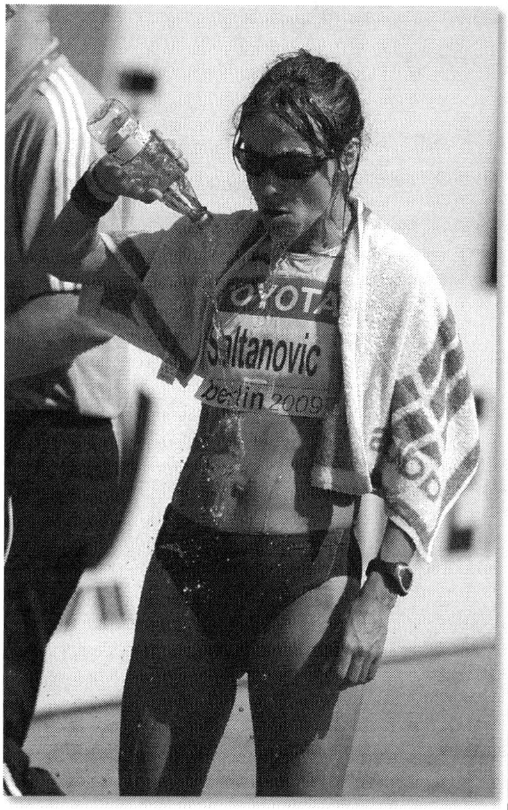

Kristina Saltanovic cooling down after finishing the World Championships

Weekly Notes

MONDAY

TUESDAY

WEDNESDAY

THURSDAY

FRIDAY

SATURDAY

SUNDAY

MONDAY	Date:	Location:	2nd workout:	
W/U Distance :	W/U Time:			
Workout Type:			Total Daily Distance:	
C/D Distance:	C/D Time:			

TUESDAY	Date:	Location:	2nd workout:	
W/U Distance :	W/U Time:			
Workout Type:			Total Daily Distance:	
C/D Distance:	C/D Time:			

WEDNESDAY	Date:	Location:	2nd workout:	
W/U Distance :	W/U Time:			
Workout Type:			Total Daily Distance:	
C/D Distance:	C/D Time:			

THURSDAY	Date:	Location:	2nd workout:	
W/U Distance :	W/U Time:			
Workout Type:			Total Daily Distance:	
C/D Distance:	C/D Time:			

FRIDAY	Date:	Location:	2nd workout:	
W/U Distance :	W/U Time:			
Workout Type:			Total Daily Distance:	
C/D Distance:	C/D Time:			

SATURDAY	Date:	Location:	2nd workout:	
W/U Distance :	W/U Time:			
Workout Type:			Total Daily Distance:	
C/D Distance:	C/D Time:			

SUNDAY	Date:	Location:	2nd workout:	
W/U Distance :	W/U Time:			
Workout Type:			Total Daily Distance:	
C/D Distance:	C/D Time:			

Total Distance for the Week:	

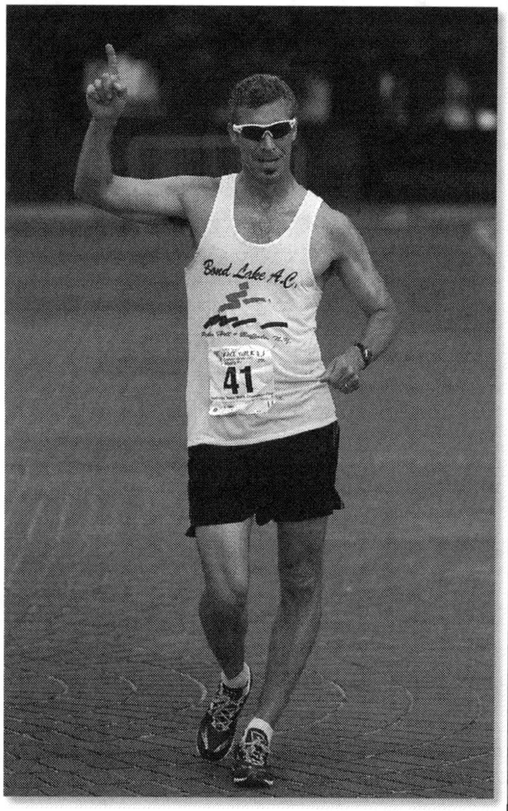

Allen James – USA
20km PR 1:24:27, 50km PR 3:55:39
16 Time National Champion, Two Time Olympian, Former US Record Holder

Weekly Notes

MONDAY

TUESDAY

WEDNESDAY

THURSDAY

FRIDAY

SATURDAY

SUNDAY

MONDAY	Date:	Location:	2nd workout:
W/U Distance :	W/U Time:		
Workout Type:			Total Daily Distance:
C/D Distance:	C/D Time:		

TUESDAY	Date:	Location:	2nd workout:
W/U Distance :	W/U Time:		
Workout Type:			Total Daily Distance:
C/D Distance:	C/D Time:		

WEDNESDAY	Date:	Location:	2nd workout:
W/U Distance :	W/U Time:		
Workout Type:			Total Daily Distance:
C/D Distance:	C/D Time:		

THURSDAY	Date:	Location:	2nd workout:
W/U Distance :	W/U Time:		
Workout Type:			Total Daily Distance:
C/D Distance:	C/D Time:		

FRIDAY	Date:	Location:	2nd workout:
W/U Distance :	W/U Time:		
Workout Type:			Total Daily Distance:
C/D Distance:	C/D Time:		

SATURDAY	Date:	Location:	2nd workout:
W/U Distance :	W/U Time:		
Workout Type:			Total Daily Distance:
C/D Distance:	C/D Time:		

SUNDAY	Date:	Location:	2nd workout:
W/U Distance :	W/U Time:		
Workout Type:			Total Daily Distance:
C/D Distance:	C/D Time:		

Total Distance for the Week:	

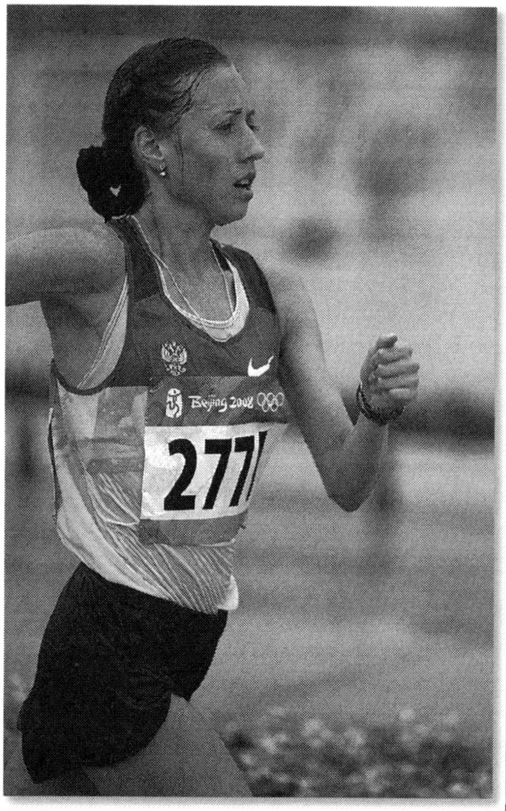

Olga Kaniskina – Russia – On her way to winning the rain-soaked 2008 Olympic Games in Beijing

Weekly Notes

MONDAY

TUESDAY

WEDNESDAY

THURSDAY

FRIDAY

SATURDAY

SUNDAY

MONDAY	Date:	Location:	2nd workout:
W/U Distance :	W/U Time:		
Workout Type:			Total Daily Distance:
C/D Distance:	C/D Time:		

TUESDAY	Date:	Location:	2nd workout:
W/U Distance :	W/U Time:		
Workout Type:			Total Daily Distance:
C/D Distance:	C/D Time:		

WEDNESDAY	Date:	Location:	2nd workout:
W/U Distance :	W/U Time:		
Workout Type:			Total Daily Distance:
C/D Distance:	C/D Time:		

THURSDAY	Date:	Location:	2nd workout:
W/U Distance :	W/U Time:		
Workout Type:			Total Daily Distance:
C/D Distance:	C/D Time:		

FRIDAY	Date:	Location:	2nd workout:
W/U Distance :	W/U Time:		
Workout Type:			Total Daily Distance:
C/D Distance:	C/D Time:		

SATURDAY	Date:	Location:	2nd workout:
W/U Distance :	W/U Time:		
Workout Type:			Total Daily Distance:
C/D Distance:	C/D Time:		

SUNDAY	Date:	Location:	2nd workout:
W/U Distance :	W/U Time:		
Workout Type:			Total Daily Distance:
C/D Distance:	C/D Time:		

Total Distance for the Week:	

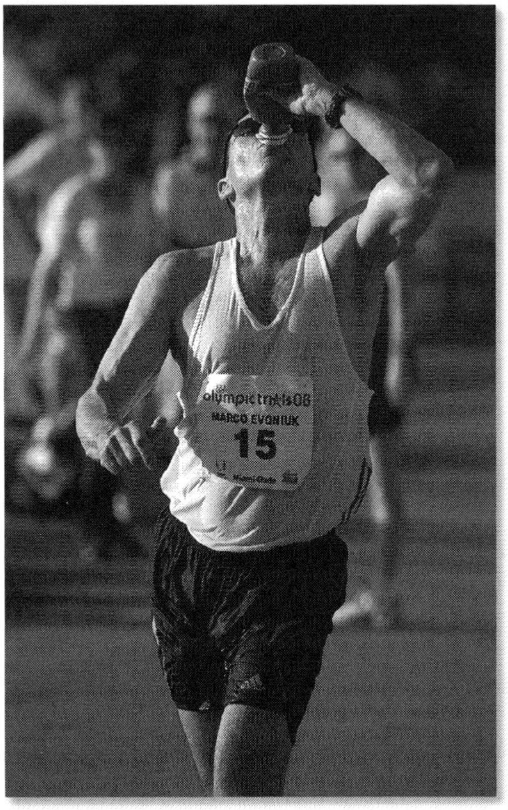

Marco Evoniuk – USA
20km PR: 1:25:23, 50km PR: 3:56:55
Four Time Olympian

Weekly Notes

MONDAY
TUESDAY
WEDNESDAY
THURSDAY
FRIDAY
SATURDAY
SUNDAY

MONDAY	Date:	Location:	2nd workout:	
W/U Distance :		W/U Time:		
Workout Type:			Total Daily Distance:	
C/D Distance:		C/D Time:		
TUESDAY	Date:	Location:	2nd workout:	
W/U Distance :		W/U Time:		
Workout Type:			Total Daily Distance:	
C/D Distance:		C/D Time:		
WEDNESDAY	Date:	Location:	2nd workout:	
W/U Distance :		W/U Time:		
Workout Type:			Total Daily Distance:	
C/D Distance:		C/D Time:		
THURSDAY	Date:	Location:	2nd workout:	
W/U Distance :		W/U Time:		
Workout Type:			Total Daily Distance:	
C/D Distance:		C/D Time:		
FRIDAY	Date:	Location:	2nd workout:	
W/U Distance :		W/U Time:		
Workout Type:			Total Daily Distance:	
C/D Distance:		C/D Time:		
SATURDAY	Date:	Location:	2nd workout:	
W/U Distance :		W/U Time:		
Workout Type:			Total Daily Distance:	
C/D Distance:		C/D Time:		
SUNDAY	Date:	Location:	2nd workout:	
W/U Distance :		W/U Time:		
Workout Type:			Total Daily Distance:	
C/D Distance:		C/D Time:		
		Total Distance for the Week:		

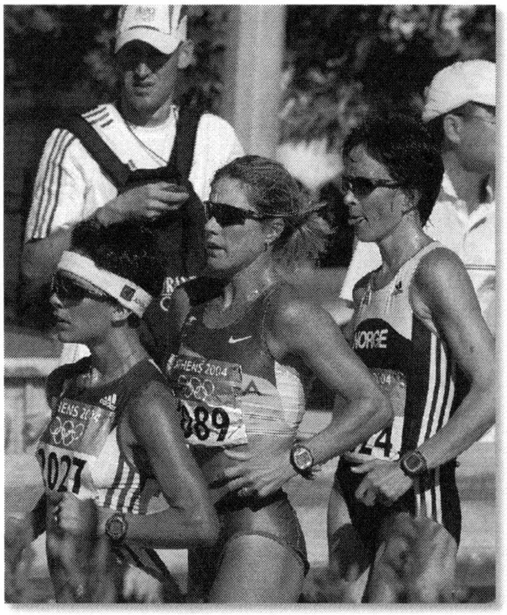

Anastasia Tsoumeléka, Jane Sayville, Kjersti Plätzer pacing together in the 2004 Olympic Games

Weekly Notes

MONDAY

TUESDAY

WEDNESDAY

THURSDAY

FRIDAY

SATURDAY

SUNDAY

MONDAY	Date:	Location:	2nd workout:	
W/U Distance :	W/U Time:			
Workout Type:			Total Daily Distance:	
C/D Distance:	C/D Time:			

TUESDAY	Date:	Location:	2nd workout:	
W/U Distance :	W/U Time:			
Workout Type:			Total Daily Distance:	
C/D Distance:	C/D Time:			

WEDNESDAY	Date:	Location:	2nd workout:	
W/U Distance :	W/U Time:			
Workout Type:			Total Daily Distance:	
C/D Distance:	C/D Time:			

THURSDAY	Date:	Location:	2nd workout:	
W/U Distance :	W/U Time:			
Workout Type:			Total Daily Distance:	
C/D Distance:	C/D Time:			

FRIDAY	Date:	Location:	2nd workout:	
W/U Distance :	W/U Time:			
Workout Type:			Total Daily Distance:	
C/D Distance:	C/D Time:			

SATURDAY	Date:	Location:	2nd workout:	
W/U Distance :	W/U Time:			
Workout Type:			Total Daily Distance:	
C/D Distance:	C/D Time:			

SUNDAY	Date:	Location:	2nd workout:	
W/U Distance :	W/U Time:			
Workout Type:			Total Daily Distance:	
C/D Distance:	C/D Time:			

Total Distance for the Week:	

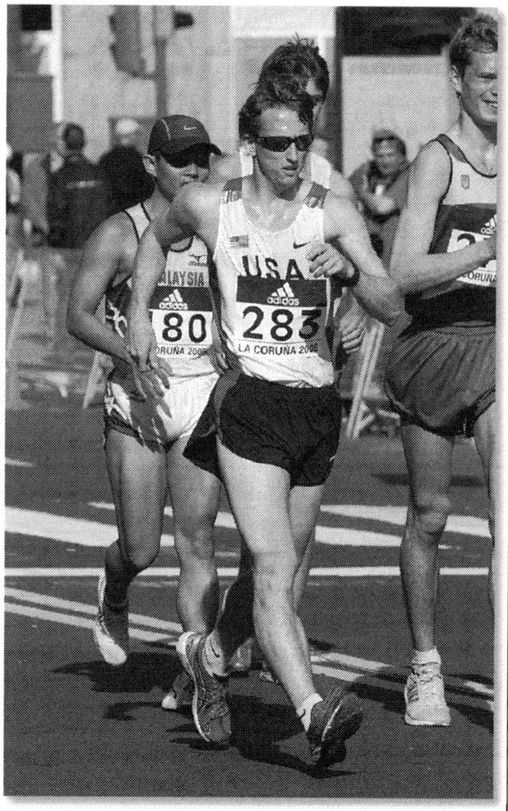

Ben Shorey – USA
20km PR: 1:27:26
Olympic Hopeful

Weekly Notes

MONDAY

TUESDAY

WEDNESDAY

THURSDAY

FRIDAY

SATURDAY

SUNDAY

MONDAY	Date:	Location:	2nd workout:
W/U Distance :	W/U Time:		
Workout Type:			
C/D Distance:	C/D Time:		Total Daily Distance:

TUESDAY	Date:	Location:	2nd workout:
W/U Distance :	W/U Time:		
Workout Type:			
C/D Distance:	C/D Time:		Total Daily Distance:

WEDNESDAY	Date:	Location:	2nd workout:
W/U Distance :	W/U Time:		
Workout Type:			
C/D Distance:	C/D Time:		Total Daily Distance:

THURSDAY	Date:	Location:	2nd workout:
W/U Distance :	W/U Time:		
Workout Type:			
C/D Distance:	C/D Time:		Total Daily Distance:

FRIDAY	Date:	Location:	2nd workout:
W/U Distance :	W/U Time:		
Workout Type:			
C/D Distance:	C/D Time:		Total Daily Distance:

SATURDAY	Date:	Location:	2nd workout:
W/U Distance :	W/U Time:		
Workout Type:			
C/D Distance:	C/D Time:		Total Daily Distance:

SUNDAY	Date:	Location:	2nd workout:
W/U Distance :	W/U Time:		
Workout Type:			
C/D Distance:	C/D Time:		Total Daily Distance:

Total Distance for the Week:	

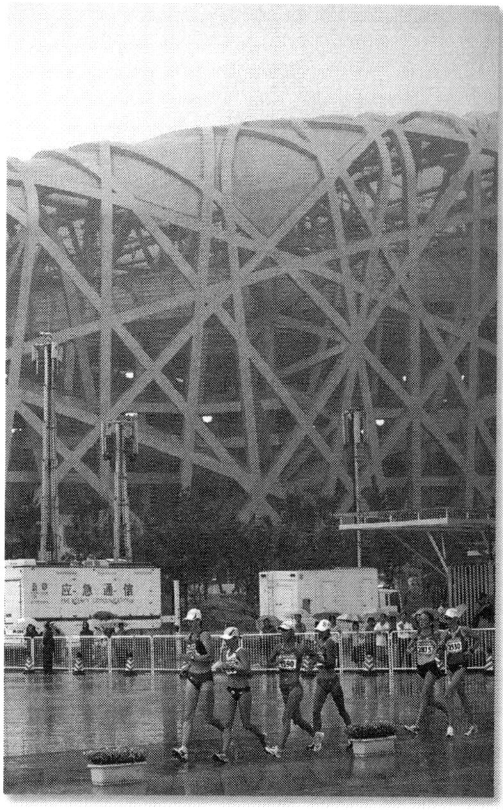

Women's Lead Pack
2008 Beijing Olympic Games

Weekly Notes

MONDAY

TUESDAY

WEDNESDAY

THURSDAY

FRIDAY

SATURDAY

SUNDAY

MONDAY	Date:	Location:	2nd workout:
W/U Distance :		W/U Time:	
Workout Type:			Total Daily Distance:
C/D Distance:		C/D Time:	

TUESDAY	Date:	Location:	2nd workout:
W/U Distance :		W/U Time:	
Workout Type:			Total Daily Distance:
C/D Distance:		C/D Time:	

WEDNESDAY	Date:	Location:	2nd workout:
W/U Distance :		W/U Time:	
Workout Type:			Total Daily Distance:
C/D Distance:		C/D Time:	

THURSDAY	Date:	Location:	2nd workout:
W/U Distance :		W/U Time:	
Workout Type:			Total Daily Distance:
C/D Distance:		C/D Time:	

FRIDAY	Date:	Location:	2nd workout:
W/U Distance :		W/U Time:	
Workout Type:			Total Daily Distance:
C/D Distance:		C/D Time:	

SATURDAY	Date:	Location:	2nd workout:
W/U Distance :		W/U Time:	
Workout Type:			Total Daily Distance:
C/D Distance:		C/D Time:	

SUNDAY	Date:	Location:	2nd workout:
W/U Distance :		W/U Time:	
Workout Type:			Total Daily Distance:
C/D Distance:		C/D Time:	

Total Distance for the Week:	

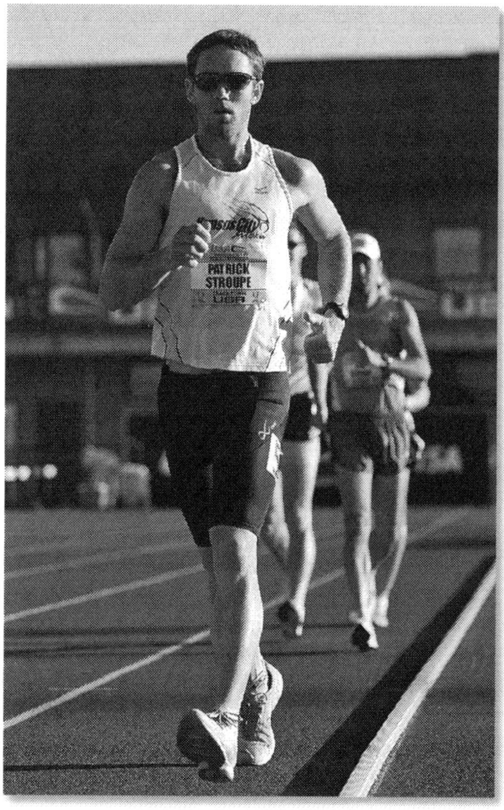

Patrick Stroupe – USA
20km PR: 1:26:41
Olympic Hopeful

Weekly Notes

MONDAY

TUESDAY

WEDNESDAY

THURSDAY

FRIDAY

SATURDAY

SUNDAY

MONDAY	Date:	Location:	2nd workout:	
W/U Distance :	W/U Time:			
Workout Type:			Total Daily Distance:	
C/D Distance:	C/D Time:			
TUESDAY	Date:	Location:	2nd workout:	
W/U Distance :	W/U Time:			
Workout Type:			Total Daily Distance:	
C/D Distance:	C/D Time:			
WEDNESDAY	Date:	Location:	2nd workout:	
W/U Distance :	W/U Time:			
Workout Type:			Total Daily Distance:	
C/D Distance:	C/D Time:			
THURSDAY	Date:	Location:	2nd workout:	
W/U Distance :	W/U Time:			
Workout Type:			Total Daily Distance:	
C/D Distance:	C/D Time:			
FRIDAY	Date:	Location:	2nd workout:	
W/U Distance :	W/U Time:			
Workout Type:			Total Daily Distance:	
C/D Distance:	C/D Time:			
SATURDAY	Date:	Location:	2nd workout:	
W/U Distance :	W/U Time:			
Workout Type:			Total Daily Distance:	
C/D Distance:	C/D Time:			
SUNDAY	Date:	Location:	2nd workout:	
W/U Distance :	W/U Time:			
Workout Type:			Total Daily Distance:	
C/D Distance:	C/D Time:			
		Total Distance for the Week:		

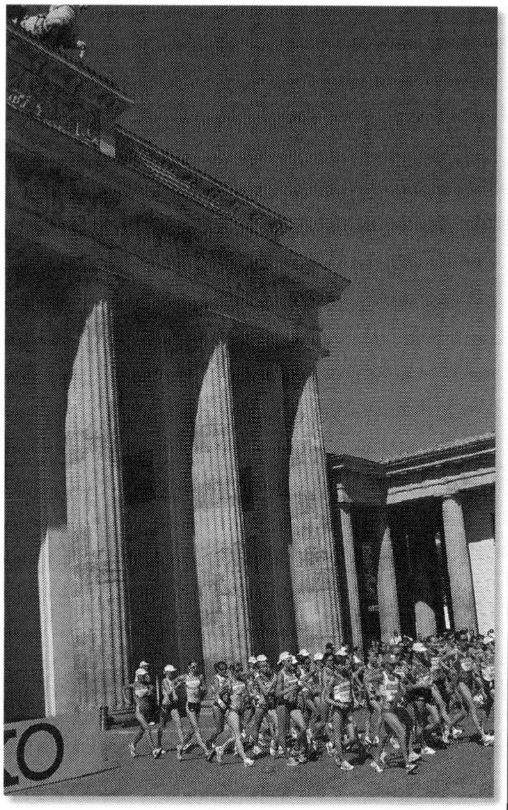

Start 20km Women's World Championships

Weekly Notes

MONDAY

TUESDAY

WEDNESDAY

THURSDAY

FRIDAY

SATURDAY

SUNDAY

MONDAY	Date:	Location:	2nd workout:
W/U Distance :	W/U Time:		
Workout Type:		Total Daily Distance:	
C/D Distance:	C/D Time:		

TUESDAY	Date:	Location:	2nd workout:
W/U Distance :	W/U Time:		
Workout Type:		Total Daily Distance:	
C/D Distance:	C/D Time:		

WEDNESDAY	Date:	Location:	2nd workout:
W/U Distance :	W/U Time:		
Workout Type:		Total Daily Distance:	
C/D Distance:	C/D Time:		

THURSDAY	Date:	Location:	2nd workout:
W/U Distance :	W/U Time:		
Workout Type:		Total Daily Distance:	
C/D Distance:	C/D Time:		

FRIDAY	Date:	Location:	2nd workout:
W/U Distance :	W/U Time:		
Workout Type:		Total Daily Distance:	
C/D Distance:	C/D Time:		

SATURDAY	Date:	Location:	2nd workout:
W/U Distance :	W/U Time:		
Workout Type:		Total Daily Distance:	
C/D Distance:	C/D Time:		

SUNDAY	Date:	Location:	2nd workout:
W/U Distance :	W/U Time:		
Workout Type:		Total Daily Distance:	
C/D Distance:	C/D Time:		

Total Distance for the Week:	

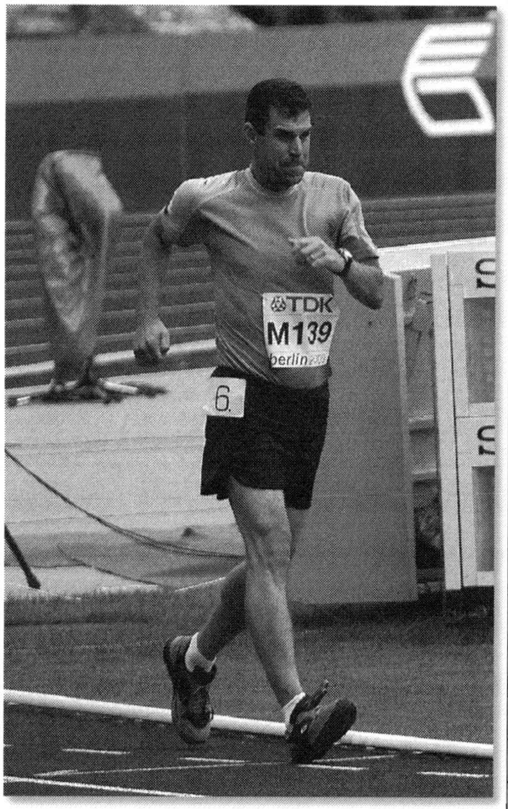

Jeff Salvage – USA
Race Walk Promoter, Writer, Competitor

Weekly Notes

MONDAY

TUESDAY

WEDNESDAY

THURSDAY

FRIDAY

SATURDAY

SUNDAY

MONDAY	Date:	Location:	2nd workout:
W/U Distance :	W/U Time:		
Workout Type:			Total Daily Distance:
C/D Distance:	C/D Time:		

TUESDAY	Date:	Location:	2nd workout:
W/U Distance :	W/U Time:		
Workout Type:			Total Daily Distance:
C/D Distance:	C/D Time:		

WEDNESDAY	Date:	Location:	2nd workout:
W/U Distance :	W/U Time:		
Workout Type:			Total Daily Distance:
C/D Distance:	C/D Time:		

THURSDAY	Date:	Location:	2nd workout:
W/U Distance :	W/U Time:		
Workout Type:			Total Daily Distance:
C/D Distance:	C/D Time:		

FRIDAY	Date:	Location:	2nd workout:
W/U Distance :	W/U Time:		
Workout Type:			Total Daily Distance:
C/D Distance:	C/D Time:		

SATURDAY	Date:	Location:	2nd workout:
W/U Distance :	W/U Time:		
Workout Type:			Total Daily Distance:
C/D Distance:	C/D Time:		

SUNDAY	Date:	Location:	2nd workout:
W/U Distance :	W/U Time:		
Workout Type:			Total Daily Distance:
C/D Distance:	C/D Time:		

Total Distance for the Week:	

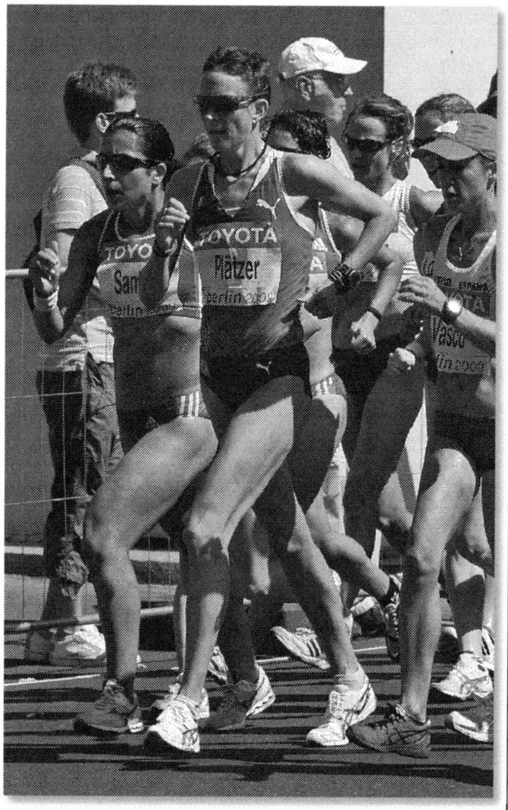

Lead Pack 20km Women's
2009 World Championships

Weekly Notes

MONDAY

TUESDAY

WEDNESDAY

THURSDAY

FRIDAY

SATURDAY

SUNDAY

MONDAY	Date:	Location:	2nd workout:	
W/U Distance :		W/U Time:		
Workout Type:				
C/D Distance:		C/D Time:	Total Daily Distance:	

TUESDAY	Date:	Location:	2nd workout:	
W/U Distance :		W/U Time:		
Workout Type:				
C/D Distance:		C/D Time:	Total Daily Distance:	

WEDNESDAY	Date:	Location:	2nd workout:	
W/U Distance :		W/U Time:		
Workout Type:				
C/D Distance:		C/D Time:	Total Daily Distance:	

THURSDAY	Date:	Location:	2nd workout:	
W/U Distance :		W/U Time:		
Workout Type:				
C/D Distance:		C/D Time:	Total Daily Distance:	

FRIDAY	Date:	Location:	2nd workout:	
W/U Distance :		W/U Time:		
Workout Type:				
C/D Distance:		C/D Time:	Total Daily Distance:	

SATURDAY	Date:	Location:	2nd workout:	
W/U Distance :		W/U Time:		
Workout Type:				
C/D Distance:		C/D Time:	Total Daily Distance:	

SUNDAY	Date:	Location:	2nd workout:	
W/U Distance :		W/U Time:		
Workout Type:				
C/D Distance:		C/D Time:	Total Daily Distance:	

Total Distance for the Week:	

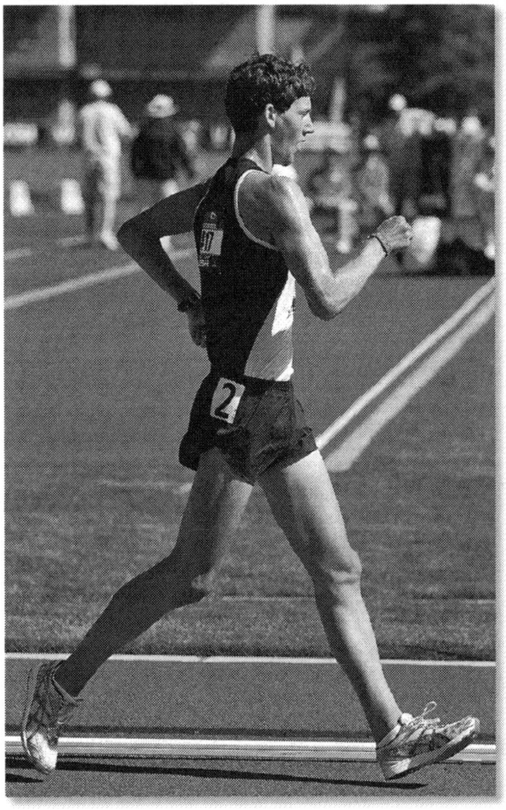

Trevor Barron – USA
10km PR: 42:22, US Jr. Record Holder
US Junior National Champion
Olympic Hopeful

Weekly Notes

MONDAY

TUESDAY

WEDNESDAY

THURSDAY

FRIDAY

SATURDAY

SUNDAY

MONDAY	Date:	Location:	2nd workout:
W/U Distance :		W/U Time:	
Workout Type:			
			Total Daily Distance:
C/D Distance:		C/D Time:	

TUESDAY	Date:	Location:	2nd workout:
W/U Distance :		W/U Time:	
Workout Type:			
			Total Daily Distance:
C/D Distance:		C/D Time:	

WEDNESDAY	Date:	Location:	2nd workout:
W/U Distance :		W/U Time:	
Workout Type:			
			Total Daily Distance:
C/D Distance:		C/D Time:	

THURSDAY	Date:	Location:	2nd workout:
W/U Distance :		W/U Time:	
Workout Type:			
			Total Daily Distance:
C/D Distance:		C/D Time:	

FRIDAY	Date:	Location:	2nd workout:
W/U Distance :		W/U Time:	
Workout Type:			
			Total Daily Distance:
C/D Distance:		C/D Time:	

SATURDAY	Date:	Location:	2nd workout:
W/U Distance :		W/U Time:	
Workout Type:			
			Total Daily Distance:
C/D Distance:		C/D Time:	

SUNDAY	Date:	Location:	2nd workout:
W/U Distance :		W/U Time:	
Workout Type:			
			Total Daily Distance:
C/D Distance:		C/D Time:	

Total Distance for the Week:	

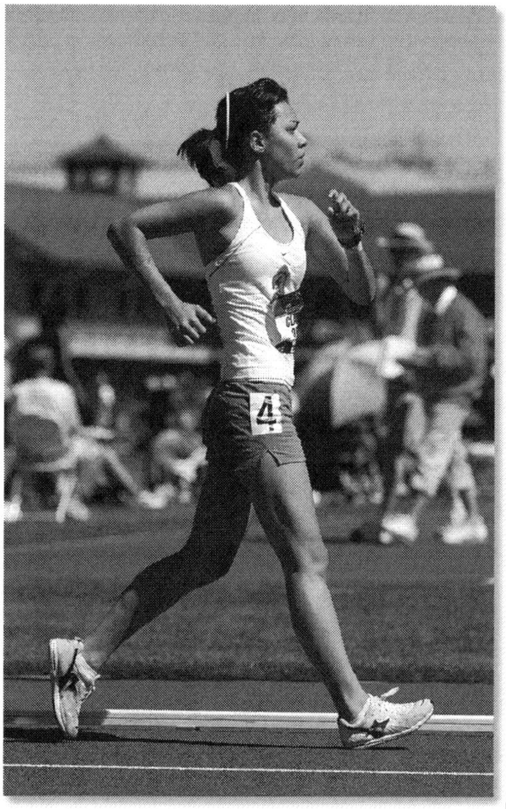

Claudia Ortiz – USA
10km PR: 57:11
US Junior Olympic Champion

Weekly Notes

MONDAY
TUESDAY
WEDNESDAY
THURSDAY
FRIDAY
SATURDAY
SUNDAY

MONDAY	Date:	Location:	2nd workout:
W/U Distance :	W/U Time:		
Workout Type:			Total Daily Distance:
C/D Distance:	C/D Time:		

TUESDAY	Date:	Location:	2nd workout:
W/U Distance :	W/U Time:		
Workout Type:			Total Daily Distance:
C/D Distance:	C/D Time:		

WEDNESDAY	Date:	Location:	2nd workout:
W/U Distance :	W/U Time:		
Workout Type:			Total Daily Distance:
C/D Distance:	C/D Time:		

THURSDAY	Date:	Location:	2nd workout:
W/U Distance :	W/U Time:		
Workout Type:			Total Daily Distance:
C/D Distance:	C/D Time:		

FRIDAY	Date:	Location:	2nd workout:
W/U Distance :	W/U Time:		
Workout Type:			Total Daily Distance:
C/D Distance:	C/D Time:		

SATURDAY	Date:	Location:	2nd workout:
W/U Distance :	W/U Time:		
Workout Type:			Total Daily Distance:
C/D Distance:	C/D Time:		

SUNDAY	Date:	Location:	2nd workout:
W/U Distance :	W/U Time:		
Workout Type:			Total Daily Distance:
C/D Distance:	C/D Time:		

Total Distance for the Week:	

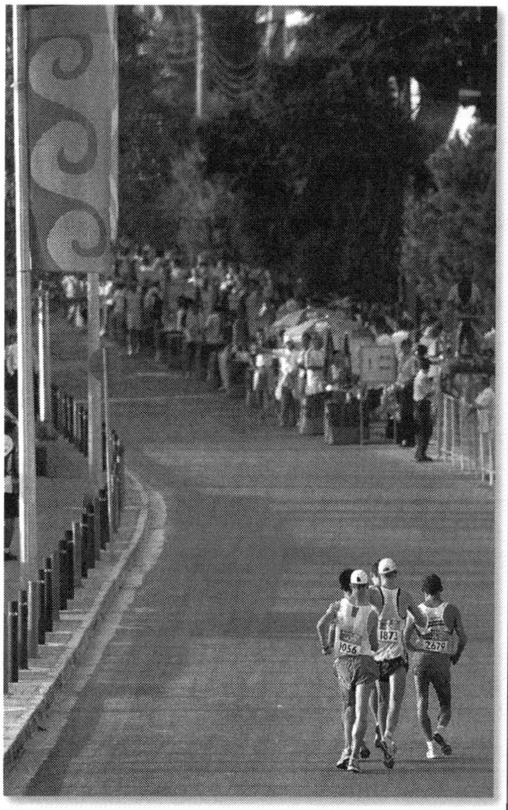

Lead Pack - Men's 50km – Athens Olympics

Weekly Notes

MONDAY

TUESDAY

WEDNESDAY

THURSDAY

FRIDAY

SATURDAY

SUNDAY

MONDAY	Date:	Location:	2nd workout:
W/U Distance :	W/U Time:		
Workout Type:			Total Daily Distance:
C/D Distance:	C/D Time:		

TUESDAY	Date:	Location:	2nd workout:
W/U Distance :	W/U Time:		
Workout Type:			Total Daily Distance:
C/D Distance:	C/D Time:		

WEDNESDAY	Date:	Location:	2nd workout:
W/U Distance :	W/U Time:		
Workout Type:			Total Daily Distance:
C/D Distance:	C/D Time:		

THURSDAY	Date:	Location:	2nd workout:
W/U Distance :	W/U Time:		
Workout Type:			Total Daily Distance:
C/D Distance:	C/D Time:		

FRIDAY	Date:	Location:	2nd workout:
W/U Distance :	W/U Time:		
Workout Type:			Total Daily Distance:
C/D Distance:	C/D Time:		

SATURDAY	Date:	Location:	2nd workout:
W/U Distance :	W/U Time:		
Workout Type:			Total Daily Distance:
C/D Distance:	C/D Time:		

SUNDAY	Date:	Location:	2nd workout:
W/U Distance :	W/U Time:		
Workout Type:			Total Daily Distance:
C/D Distance:	C/D Time:		

Total Distance for the Week:	

Race Record

Date:	Distance:	Name:
Rank:	Time:	Location:
Date:	Distance:	Name:
Rank:	Time:	Location:
Date:	Distance:	Name:
Rank:	Time:	Location:
Date:	Distance:	Name:
Rank:	Time:	Location:
Date:	Distance:	Name:
Rank:	Time:	Location:
Date:	Distance:	Name:
Rank:	Time:	Location:
Date:	Distance:	Name:
Rank:	Time:	Location:

Race Record

Date:	**Distance:**	**Name:**
Rank:	**Time:**	**Location:**
Date:	**Distance:**	**Name:**
Rank:	**Time:**	**Location:**
Date:	**Distance:**	**Name:**
Rank:	**Time:**	**Location:**
Date:	**Distance:**	**Name:**
Rank:	**Time:**	**Location:**
Date:	**Distance:**	**Name:**
Rank:	**Time:**	**Location:**
Date:	**Distance:**	**Name:**
Rank:	**Time:**	**Location:**
Date:	**Distance:**	**Name:**
Rank:	**Time:**	**Location:**

Race Record

Date:	**Distance:**	**Name:**
Rank:	**Time:**	**Location:**
Date:	**Distance:**	**Name:**
Rank:	**Time:**	**Location:**
Date:	**Distance:**	**Name:**
Rank:	**Time:**	**Location:**
Date:	**Distance:**	**Name:**
Rank:	**Time:**	**Location:**
Date:	**Distance:**	**Name:**
Rank:	**Time:**	**Location:**
Date:	**Distance:**	**Name:**
Rank:	**Time:**	**Location:**
Date:	**Distance:**	**Name:**
Rank:	**Time:**	**Location:**

Race Record

Date:	Distance:	Name:
Rank:	Time:	Location:
Date:	Distance:	Name:
Rank:	Time:	Location:
Date:	Distance:	Name:
Rank:	Time:	Location:
Date:	Distance:	Name:
Rank:	Time:	Location:
Date:	Distance:	Name:
Rank:	Time:	Location:
Date:	Distance:	Name:
Rank:	Time:	Location:
Date:	Distance:	Name:
Rank:	Time:	Location:

Total Distance for Each Month

Month	Distance
January	
February	
March	
April	
May	
June	
July	
August	
September	
October	
November	
December	
Yearly Total	

Other Yearly Totals

Total # of Training Days:	**Average Distance Per Training Day:**
Total # of Days Off:	**Average Monthly Distance:**

Personal Record Progression

Indoor Competition

1 mile	3000 M	5000M

Outdoor Competition

1 mile	3KM	5KM

Personal Record Progression

Outdoor Competition (continued)

10KM	15KM	20KM

30KM	40KM	50KM

Additional Publications by Walking Promotions

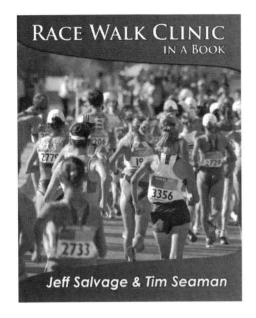

America's premier team of clinicians Jeff Salvage and Tim Seaman's ***Race Walk Clinic — in a Book*** beautifully illustrates textbook techniques while it catalogs typical mistakes race walkers make that can rob them of a legal race and speed. It explains why these problems exist and prescribes critical solutions to correct them. If you are ready to improve your race walking style and step up to the next level, then pick up ***Race Walk Clinic - in a Book*** today.

Our approach in *Race Walk Clinic — in a Book* is to pick up where other training materials leave off. We start by grounding our discussion with a review of correct race walking technique, but do not focus on the many aspects of technique that you can do incorrectly. We then divide race walking technique problems into broad categories, starting with issues of legality and then separating technique issues into categories such as hip, leg, arm, and posture problems.

For each category we illustrate the problem with photographs of either elite race walkers or (for beginner problems) staged images. We then offer remediation in two forms: exercises, drills, and stretches to improve your style, and mental cues to guide your focus while race walking.Within the educational material presented, we've interspersed "Tales from the Track," a unique collection of unique stories in which great race walkers from the U.S. and around the world retell some of their most memorable experiences.

Order from www.racewalk.com or www.racewalkclinic.com for $23.95 + S&H

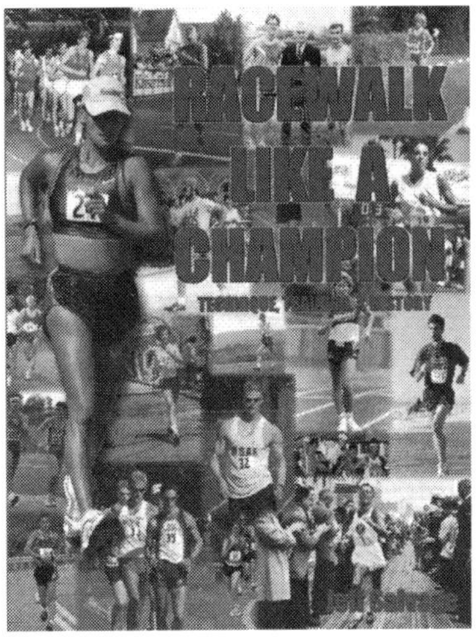

Printed with 8 1/2 x 11 full-color pages, ***Race Walk Like a Champion*** is the single best compilation of information on the technique, training, and history of race walking. It combines approximately 400 photographs with charts and diagrams to explain every detail of race walking.

Race Walk Like a Champion starts with a thorough explanation of how to select race walking shoes and warmup; it then describes every aspect of race walking technique, judging, and training philosophy in extensive detail. Other chapters include stretching, racing, strength training, mental preparation, injury treatment, and nutrition. ***Race Walk Like a Champion*** also includes a comprehensive chapter on the history of American race walking. Each era of walking is described with an introduction and biographies of that period's greats.

Order from www.racewalk.com for $23.95 + S&H

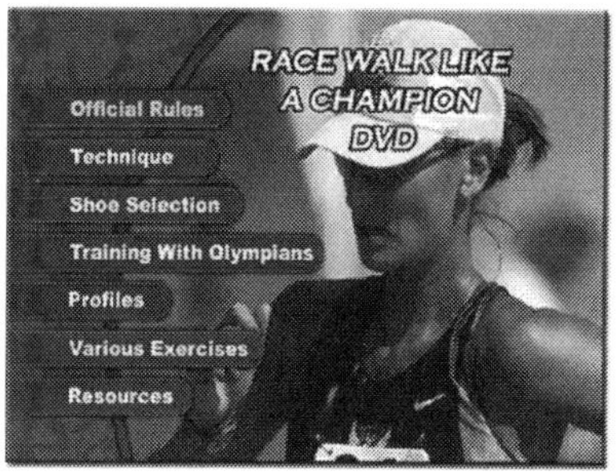

The *Race Walk Like a Champion* companion DVD/CD brings the descriptions from the book to life while explaining all aspects of race walking in DVD-quality video. However, the benefits of the DVD format do not end there; the interactivity makes it a coach in a box. Its friendly menus allow you to watch exactly the section you wish, over and over, with no rewinding! Have a technique problem? Just drill down through the interactive menus and your everpresent coach is there to assist.

Order from www.racewalk.com for $49.95 + S&H

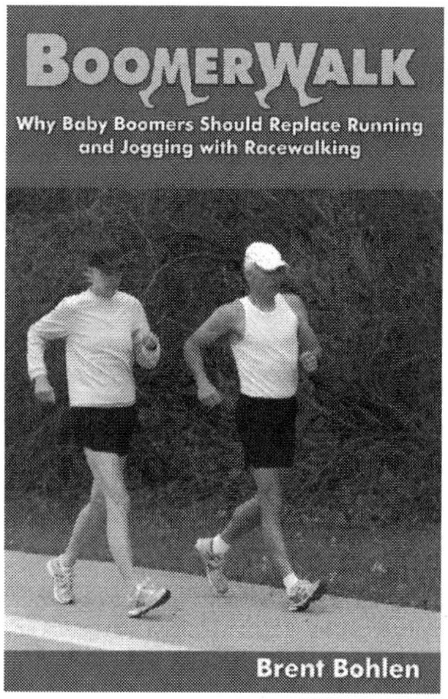

If you are reading this page, you clearly are already interested in race walking and have a strong knowledge of the sport. How about inspiring one of the 75 million baby boomers who need to learn about our great sport? *BoomerWalk* is written to inspire a wide range of people to become race walkers. It is a great summary of basic technique that motivates readers to get off the couch and start race walking. Author Brent Bohlen relates his experience in discovering the sport of race walking at a time in his life when his aging knees no longer could take the pounding of his four-decade love of basketball. Race walking provided him the cardiovascular fitness he needed, the competition he wanted, and the kindness his knees demanded. Once he convinces you to take up race walking, whether for fitness or for competition, Bohlen provides the basics of race walking technique to get you off on the right foot. You can begin race walking right away with no special equipment.

Order from www.BoomerWalk.com, www.racewalk.com, or www.amazon.com for $15.95 + S&H.

6235091R0

Made in the USA
Charleston, SC
30 September 2010